Becoming an Alzheimer's Caregiver

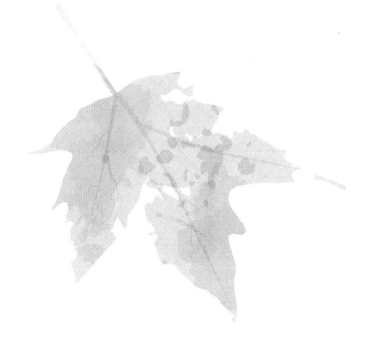

Becoming an Alzheimer's Caregiver

What I Learned from Caring for My Mom

by Amy Neuzil

Contents

Foreword

"I'm sorry, but you have dementia caused by Alzheimer's disease." As terrifying as many find these words to be, most people don't fully understand dementia or its many causes. Nonetheless, they believe there is nothing that can be done. But is that true?

In fact, there are many things that can be done for those affected by dementia, as well as for their families. Although most dementias are progressive and impact life, this does not mean that a meaningful life is over. There are typically years of life ahead, and these can be good years with the right guidance and resources. Dementia does not mean that there are no more times of joy to experience, no more dreams to dream, and no more good memories to reflect upon. It does mean that those affected by dementia will need to accept that, in the future, they will require a caregiving team focused on promoting their independence and function, while securing their safety at the same time.

The diagnosis of dementia and its causes is relatively straightforward. A careful interview of patient and family can yield the areas of cognition that have been affected, resulting in loss of independence. Often memory and decision making are two such domains. Dementia is an effect. But what is the cause? The cause is a disease in the brain. There are dozens of diseases that can impair the processes of the brain and result in dementia, the most common being Alzheimer's disease, frontotemporal lobar degeneration, Lewy body disease, and vascular disease. Thus, there are actually two questions: what is the process occurring in the brain, and what is its impact on life?

However, the real challenge comes after the diagnosis. This is when care planning for the overall health and daily needs of affected individuals becomes crucial. Part of this plan must include the needs and availability of the caregivers. I have the opportunity to meet with patients and families on a daily basis and our greatest challenge is in finding solutions for the ongoing care needs resulting from dementia. We explore the options and pursue a care plan to address those concerns.

During the first years of this third millennium, we have seen a significant decline in mortality associated with heart disease and stroke, as well as with breast and prostate cancers. However, we have seen no such decline in deaths caused by Alzheimer's disease. Currently, we are seeing rapid increases in both public awareness and research funding. The great hope is that, over the coming years, we will discover treatments that will increasingly slow the progression of this disease. At some point, we will be able to arrest the development of Alzheimer's disease and ultimately prevent it. However, even if that occurred tomorrow, there would still be affected individuals who would require the love and care of others for many years. On top of this is the fact that there are many other diseases in the brain that can cause dementia. These will all likely require different treatments to prevent the onset of dementia. Until these hoped for therapies are found, many families will be faced with the challenges of caregiving for their loved ones with dementia.

The internet has forever changed the way that we obtain information. However, that information is of variable quality, and it is important to find material that is accurate. The trouble that many caregivers run into is that there is typically little direction in navigating the complex information related to caregiving needs, financial needs, legal needs, and the community resources that are frequently required. It can be difficult to find a roadmap that provides needed guidance. Amy has provided us with such a map.

In addition to a reliable guide and source of information, we need the insights of those who have walked the path before us. Such wisdom comes only from the experience of caring for someone with dementia.

Dementia is not the life that individuals or their families would choose, but it is a life that can be meaningful. It is a common myth that there is nothing you can do. In this book, you will find many personal and touching stories showing that, in fact, there is a great deal that you can do. Read on.

—*Robert S. Keyes, MD, PhD*
The Christ Hospital Health and Aging Center
Cincinnati, Ohio

Acknowledgments

First and foremost, thank you to my editors Joan Liebmann-Smith, PhD and Monica Payson, who worked with me at different stages of the editing process. Both Joan and Monica had personal experiences of losing someone special to dementia, and both made this book better because of their writing and editing talents, attention to detail, gentle guidance, unique insights, and compassionate voices.

I was so fortunate to hear Dr. Robert Keyes speak at an Alzheimer's Association-sponsored event not long after Mom had moved into the nursing home. I was impressed not only with his knowledge of Alzheimer's dementia but with his ability to present it so tenderly to an auditorium full of Alzheimer's caregivers. Dr. Keyes, I am so grateful that you agreed to volunteer your expert voice to this project and that your thoughts and reflections are the first words read by the reader.

My family and I have been blessed to encounter so many people through the years who provide such merciful and tender care to this vulnerable and growing population. They need to be acknowledged.

To the doctors, nurses, and other healthcare professionals and researchers who are caring for those with Alzheimer's or searching for effective treatments and a cure, thank you so much. I am humbled by your dedication.

To those who never met Mom but profoundly influenced her care through their gentle direction, you have my deepest appreciation: Linda from A Place for Mom and the counselors at the Greater Cincinnati Chapter of the Alzheimer's Association.

My heartfelt gratitude to those who have cared so compassionately for Mom these past several years: the staff at the University of Cincinnati Medical Center Memory Disorders Center and the staff at Western Hills Mercy Hospital.

Special thanks to the staff at Meadowbrook Care Center in Cincinnati, Ohio. Mom came to you following a period of immense stress and uncertainty, especially for Mom, but for the rest of the family as well. You give us peace of mind by taking such great care of her. And you take the time to see past her dementia, to learn about who she was, who she still is. Thank you so very much.

Finally, to my husband who encouraged and supported me every step of the way by reminding me that I was bound to help someone. Thanks so much, Paul.

Abbreviations

AARP	American Association of Retired Persons
ADEAR	Alzheimer's Disease Education and Referral Center
AGS	American Geriatrics Society
AOTA	American Occupational Therapy Association
CDC	Centers for Disease Control and Prevention
FDA	Food and Drug Administration
NADSA	National Adult Day Services Association
NHPCO	National Hospice and Palliative Care Organization
NHTSA	National Highway Traffic Safety Administration
NIA	National Institute on Aging
NIH	National Institutes of Health

Introduction

I first noticed my mom's memory struggles in 2001. She was diagnosed with **mild cognitive impairment** two years later, and in 2006 that diagnosis was changed to **Alzheimer's disease.**

Mom was living at home in Cincinnati with my dad. My younger sister Mary and I each lived a short fifteen-minute drive from our parents' house, which was very convenient because our caregiving commitment increased tremendously as Mom's **dementia** worsened. My youngest sister, Barb, who had lived across the country and visited when she could, was able to move back home when Mom was at her worst. While it was a blessing to have Barb back in Cincinnati to join in as a caregiver and decision-maker, I believe the most valuable thing Barb had to offer was her perspective. She was able to view the rapidly declining circumstances at my parents' house more clearly and objectively than Dad, Mary, or I.

While Dad assumed the bulk of the responsibilities of being Mom's primary caregiver, my two sisters and I were also very involved in her care until 2012 when she was moved to a nursing home. The months leading up to that move felt like we were perpetually residing in the twilight zone as **sundowning**

behaviors took hold of Mom and prevented Dad, most nota-
bly, from getting the daily rest he needed to face his caregiving
duties the next day. If Mom couldn't sleep because her confusion led to anxiety and then her anxiety led to agitation and
anger, Dad couldn't sleep either because he feared for Mom's
safety when she was so unsettled. So he stayed up with Mom,
following her from room to room to keep a watchful eye on
her. Obviously, that couldn't be maintained indefinitely.

Both Mary and I are registered nurses and, upon reflection,
that was both a help and a hindrance when caring for Mom.
Undoubtedly our nursing education and experience helped
us better understand the terminology used by her doctors and
nurses. Whether it was the medications prescribed for her or
the complex changes that were taking place in her brain, we
were able to understand intellectually the resultant decline
in Mom's language skills, the behaviors that surfaced, and her
gradual descent into dementia.

However, as Mom worsened, Mary and I struggled to
acknowledge when she had reached the point when she
needed different care than we could provide for her at home.
That realization was difficult for each member of my family,
and I believe my Dad's heart did break having to make the
decision to move Mom to a nursing home. And while living
out of town had insulated Barb from the day-to-day caregiving
stress, it was difficult for her too. But I think the move stung in
a more personal way for Mary and me because, as nurses, we
naturally viewed ourselves as caregivers.

Mom's been living in the nursing home for five years now.
However, the nursing home we initially chose for Mom, where
she spent several weeks in early 2012, is not the one where she
lives now. That first nursing home experience was negative
for every member of my family, but it ended up serving a very
important purpose. When we began our search for another
nursing home just weeks into Mom's move into the first, our

priorities were clarified: we were more observant while touring prospective homes, we were better prepared with pertinent questions for nursing home staff members, and we were better prepared to share pertinent information regarding Mom's health, especially as it related to her Alzheimer's disease.

Mom acknowledged to me only once in all those years that she was aware of having Alzheimer's disease. Her dad had died in 1981 with symptoms that were similar in so many ways to Mom's, and she truly feared developing it herself. However, she refused to discuss it, even with her family. It wasn't until early 2012 that we accidentally discovered, hidden away, a yellow legal pad that Mom used to journal her feelings about the changes going on inside of her. In grief, she acknowledged her disease, voiced her fears and resolutely vowed to beat it.

It's been such a long road with Mom, and we've learned a lot about caring for someone with Alzheimer's disease. The advice and education we received from the Alzheimer's Association and other caregiving organizations and publications armed us with strategies to make caregiving less stressful. However, sometimes the best teachers were the mistakes we made because they forced us to look at a caregiving issue from a different angle. I would like to share with you what we learned through this journey of being Mom's caregivers. It's my sincerest wish that this book offer you guidance, support, and hope.

One

Alzheimer's Disease: The Basics

A Brief History of the Disease

In 1906, a German physician gave a lecture in which he described a patient who presented with a group of symptoms that included problems with memory, reading and writing, disorientation, cognitive decline, and **hallucinations**. This case was fascinating for a couple of reasons. First, the group of symptoms was more commonly associated with the elderly, but the patient was fifty-five years old. And second, the brain autopsy findings following her death showed several abnormalities:

- Loss of brain mass (the physical size was smaller than that of a healthy brain)
- The **cerebral cortex** was thinner than normal[1]

In addition, there was evidence of **senile plaques,** previously seen only in elderly people.[2] (Romanian born neuroscientist Georges Marinesco and French pathologist Paul Blocz gave the first account of senile plaques. It's interesting to note that they didn't associate these plaques with dementia as their examination was limited to nine deceased patients with histories of epilepsy.)[3] There was also evidence of **neurofibrillary tangles.** The physician was able to identify these nerve tangles because of a new technique in microscopic staining. These nerve tangles had never been described before.[4]

Today, the definitive diagnosis of Alzheimer's disease is not made until after death when an autopsy is performed. It's worth noting that the pathological diagnosis (examination of brain tissue at autopsy) of Alzheimer's disease is based largely on the same methods used in 1906.[5]

The physician who first described this disease was Dr. Aloysius *Alois* Alzheimer, a psychiatrist and neuropathologist. Who was the patient who, unknowingly, served as a case study for a gifted physician whose name was given to the disease he helped to identify? The patient was Auguste Deter. There is very little information available about Ms. Deter. However, a comment she made to her physician seems prophetic for the millions affected by this disease: "I've lost myself."[6]

Alzheimer's Disease Timeline

Since 1906, several events are worth mentioning due to their importance in the historical timeline of this disease:

1910   The term *Alzheimer's disease* first appears in print in Dr. Emil Kraepelin's book, *Compendium der Psychiatrie*, 8th ed.[7]

1960s   The medical community formally recognizes Alzheimer's as a disease and not a normal part of aging.[8]

1968   The first substantiated measurement scale is developed by researchers to assess cognitive and functional decline in older adults.[9]

1974   The National Institute on Aging (NIA) is founded and becomes the leading federal agency supporting Alzheimer's disease research.[10]

1976   Alzheimer's disease is recognized as the most common form of dementia as published in *Archives of Neurology* by neurologist Robert Katzman.[11]

1980   The Alzheimer's Association is formed.

1984   The first Alzheimer's disease centers are formed.[12]

1986   The Alzheimer's Disease Education and Referral (ADEAR) Center, through the NIA, begins conducting research and distributing information about Alzheimer's disease to health professionals, patients and their families, and the general public.[13]

1987   Clinical trials begin on the first drug explicitly targeting Alzheimer's disease symptoms.[14]

1993   The first Food and Drug Administration (FDA) approved medication (tacrine) is put on the market to treat cognitive symptoms of the disease.[15]

2010   Alzheimer's disease becomes the sixth leading cause of death in the United States.[16]

2017   The total estimated Alzheimer's disease research expenditure reaches $910 million.[17]

Alzheimer's Disease Terminology

Below is a short glossary of medical terms commonly used when discussing Alzheimer's disease. These terms are used throughout this book and are useful when talking to your loved one's physicians and other medical professionals. (For a more comprehensive glossary of Alzheimer's disease terms,

go to: my.clevelandclinic.org/health/diseases_conditions/
hic_Alzheimers_and_Dementia_Overview/hic_Alzheimers_
Disease_Glossary_of_Terms.)

Alzheimer's disease: An incurable disease in which nerve cells in the brain deteriorate and brain matter becomes smaller. As a result, thinking, behavior, and memory are impaired.[18]

Amyloid: A protein found in the brains of people with Alzheimer's disease. It builds up into *plaque* or *tangles.*[19]

Clinical trial: A research study involving humans that rigorously tests safety, side effects, and how well a medication or behavioral treatment works.[20]

Cognitive abilities: Perception, reasoning, judgment, acts of creativity, comprehension, memory, and learning are examples.[21]

Cueing: The practice of providing clues, hints or suggestions, or prompts to assist a person with memory loss.[22]

Dementia: Is not a disease unto itself but a term that describes a group of symptoms such as changes in mood, behavior and personality, as well as impaired thinking, memory, and reasoning that interfere with a person's day-to-day functioning.[23]

Drug Trials:
   Phase I – Researchers test a new drug or treatment in a small group of people (twenty to eighty) for the first time to evaluate its safety, determine a safe dosage range, and identify side effects.
   Phase II – The drug or treatment is given to a larger group of people (several hundred) to see if it's effective and to further evaluate its safety.
   Phase III – The drug or treatment is given to

large groups of people (several hundred to several thousand) to confirm its effectiveness, monitor side effects, compare it to commonly used treatments, and collect information that will allow the drug or treatment to be used safely. [24]

Early-onset Alzheimer's disease: Diagnosed before the age of sixty-five. A small percentage of those diagnosed with early-onset Alzheimer's disease have a rare gene that directly causes Alzheimer's, known as *familial Alzheimer's disease.*[25]

Hoarding: The act of collecting items and hiding or storing them away.[26]

Mild cognitive impairment: More severe than the expected cognitive decline of normal aging, but less severe than dementia. It might be noticeable to family and close friends, but is usually not severe enough to interfere with daily activities.[27]

Mini-mental state examination: Short-term memory, long-term memory, orientation, writing, and language are cognitive skills that are measured in this mental status exam.[28]

Neurofibrillary tangles: Inside nerve cells, fragments of twisted protein (tau protein) accumulate.[29]

Neuropsychological testing: Language, visual-perceptual skills, memory, attention, problem solving, and reasoning are tested to evaluate brain function and a person's capabilities.[30]

Senile plaques: Also known as beta-amyloid, which is a protein fragment that builds up between nerve cells.[31]

Rummaging: Searching through places where things are stored (for example, cabinets, drawers, closets, or the refrigerator).[32]

Sundowning/sundown syndrome: Beginning in the late afternoon and into the night, many people with Alzheimer's disease experience sundowning symptoms, which include agitation, pacing, irritability, and disorientation.[33]

Conclusion

In the next chapter, I'll discuss the process you and your loved one might experience as you begin searching for a reason for their memory difficulties. When my mom was evaluated, she presented a tough exterior. Her attitude was almost defiant. However, I could tell by the look in her eyes how frightened she was, though she wouldn't or couldn't admit it to anyone. This can be a scary time for your loved one. It's likely they are aware of the memory struggles that bring them to the doctor for evaluation. It's also quite possible your loved one has tried to manage this issue on their own for some time, before it became obvious to you that a problem even existed. As a future caregiver, take it one step at a time and be mindful to tend not only to your loved one's feelings but to yours as well.

Resources

In many cases, the additional resources I've included in each chapter provide similar information. However, I've discovered through this journey that each source might present the information a bit differently. Sometimes, those subtle differences in presentation are all you need to find something valuable to use in your unique situation.

General Information on Alzheimer's Disease

▶ **The Alzheimer's Association** 1-800-272-3900
A good place to start for gaining a background on Alzheimer's disease as well as for researching specific topics as your loved one's disease progresses.
www.alz.org

▶ **ADEAR (The Alzheimer's Disease Education and Referral Center)**
Information on Alzheimer's disease basics as well as information on causes, symptoms, and treatment.
www.nia.nih.gov/alzheimers

▶ **Family Caregiver Alliance**
Information on Alzheimer's disease, dementia, and mild cognitive impairment in a fact and tip sheet format.
www.caregiver.org/resources-health-issue-or-condition

▶ **Cleveland Clinic**
This glossary of terms provides you with an extensive list of pertinent terminology related to Alzheimer's disease.
my.clevelandclinic.org/health/articles/alzheimers-disease-glossary-of-terms

▶ *The Alzheimer's Project* (video)
HBO's *The Alzheimer's Project* presents a series of videos on many aspects of Alzheimer's disease of interest to family and caregivers.
www.hbo.com/alzheimers/index.html

▶ *The Forgetting: A Portrait of Alzheimer's* (video)
PBS's Emmy award-winning documentary based on the best-selling book by David Shenk.
www.pbs.org/program/forgetting/

Two

Getting a Diagnosis

Warning Signs

My mother began experiencing mild memory problems about two years before she was diagnosed with mild cognitive impairment. What I mean by *mild memory problems* is that she would repeat herself occasionally. For example, she might ask the same question or tell me the same story a few times per week. Looking back, I'm surprised that I even noticed it except for the fact that Mom was fearful of developing Alzheimer's disease, which I think stemmed from her dad having had dementia the last few years of his life. Mom expressed her concern to me countless times during the twenty years between her dad's death and the onset of her own memory problems.

When Mom was diagnosed with mild cognitive impairment in 2003, we were told that she had approximately a 60 percent chance of it advancing from mild cognitive impairment to Alzheimer's disease. As I write this now, "[r]esearch has shown that individuals with mild cognitive impairment have a significantly increased risk of developing Alzheimer's disease within a few years."[1]

That statement proved true in my mom's case. From the time she was diagnosed with mild cognitive impairment to the change in diagnosis to dementia of the Alzheimer's type, three years had passed. While we were saddened by this news, neither my dad, my sisters, nor I were surprised by the changed diagnosis. Mom's cognitive abilities were declining slowly, but declining nonetheless.

Following is a list from the Alzheimer's Association of warning signs that can help you determine if your loved one might be in the early stages of Alzheimer's disease. If your loved one is experiencing some or all of these symptoms, it might be time to get a professional evaluation.

Ten Warning Signs of Alzheimer's Disease[2]
- Memory loss that disrupts daily life
- Challenges in planning or solving problems
- Difficulty completing familiar tasks at home, at work, or at leisure
- Confusion with time or place
- Trouble understanding visual images and spatial relationships
- New problems with words in speaking or writing
- Misplacing things and losing the ability to retrace steps
- Decreased or poor judgment
- Withdrawal from work or social activities
- Changes in mood and personality

Getting an accurate diagnosis can be a long process. Because there are other conditions that can cause symptoms of dementia, the doctor will want to look at all possible causes in order to render an accurate diagnosis.

Preparing for the Doctor's Appointment

Going to the doctor for an evaluation can be extremely anxiety producing for both you and your loved one. Whether you are a caregiver, a concerned family member, or a friend, I recommend having the following list answered to the best of your ability and in written form before you go to the doctor. Having pertinent health information written down ahead of time will hopefully decrease some of the stress associated with a doctor visit. In addition, the history you provide is vital information for the doctor. During the visit, the doctor is likely to direct these questions to your loved one, but it's important that you correct any misinformation as well as provide any important additional information, observations, concerns that you have thought about beforehand.

Information to Have Written Down Before Getting an Evaluation

- What is the main reason for visiting the doctor today?
- What memory changes or difficulty in thinking clearly have you noticed? When did you first notice these changes?
- What activities, if any, are you struggling with that have never been a problem for you in the past?
- What medications do you currently take (including dosage and frequency)?
- Do you take your medication without assistance?
- If you are allergic to any medications, what are they and how do they affect you?
- What environmental, food, or other allergies do you have?
- Are you a smoker? If yes, how many cigarettes/packs per day?
- Do you drink alcohol? If yes, how many drinks per day? Per week?
- Do you have any dietary restrictions (e.g., low sodium, low fat, etc.)?
- Do you exercise regularly? How often and what kind of exercise?

- Do you work or volunteer outside the home? If yes, what kind of work and how many hours per day? Per week?
- What time do you typically wake in the morning?
- What time do you typically go to bed at night?
- If you wake up during the night, how often?
- Do you take naps during the day? If so, how many and for how long?
- Do you plan and prepare your own meals?
- Do you grocery shop by yourself or with assistance?
- Do you have assistance with day-to-day housekeeping duties? Explain.
- What activities, if any, do you participate in outside your home and how often? Daily? Weekly?
- Do you drive? If so, how often and how far from home? Do you need help with hygiene (e.g., brushing hair and teeth, bathing, dressing in appropriate clothing)? If yes, how much help do you need (cueing, assistance, or total care)?

The answers to these questions will change as time passes. For example, when my mom visited her doctor for the first time to discuss her memory issues, most of these questions were not relevant. The only complaint she had was a decline in her short-term memory. She was still running the household, paying the bills, cooking, cleaning, and driving independently. However, as time passed and her cognitive abilities declined, it was important to provide honest answers to these questions both to provide accurate information to Mom's doctors and to re-evaluate and plan for her increasing needs.

Further Tests Your Doctor Might Recommend

Following your loved one's initial assessment, the doctor might order further tests to aid in establishing a diagnosis.

Following is a list of tests and studies your doctor might recommend after seeing you and your loved one in the office:

- Thorough medical history and physical exam
- Laboratory tests
- Neurological exam
- Mini-Mental State Examination
- Neuropsychological assessment/neurocognitive testing
- Brain imaging studies (**MRI, CAT scan, PET scan**)
- Alzheimer's Disease Specialists

Alzheimer's Disease Specialists

There might be a number of healthcare professionals involved in your loved one's care during the process of getting a diagnosis and from that point forward. At different points in your loved one's diagnosis and treatment you might work with primary care physicians, neurologists, psychologists, geriatricians, and nurse practitioners.

In my mom's case, there were several physicians involved. The first doctor to evaluate her was her primary care physician, an internist. He promptly referred her to a neurologist, who was trained in more sophisticated testing. During that first visit with the neurologist, Mom demonstrated enough of an impairment during the brief cognitive testing that he recommended two things. The first was an MRI to rule out a stroke or other abnormality of the brain. When the results of the MRI proved to be normal, he then recommended neurocognitive testing to evaluate the extent of her cognitive impairment.

For the neurocognitive testing, my mother saw a psychologist. It took three months from the time Mom first saw her primary care physician to when she saw the psychologist for neurocognitive testing. It was then that she was diagnosed with mild cognitive impairment. After that she only saw the psychologist once a year for repeated testing to monitor changes in her cognitive function. When he finally made the diagnosis of dementia of the Alzheimer's type, Mom told us that she would never see that doctor again. After all, he had given her the diagnosis she most feared. She never did see him again but not because of her refusal. We appreciated the psychologist's competent and compassionate care, but we felt that Mom had crossed over from a diagnosis that had a chance of remaining somewhat stable and nonprogressive to one whose very nature was progressive. For that reason, we needed to adjust our game plan.

Four years after Mom was diagnosed with Alzheimer's disease, she was referred to a neurologist in a memory disorders center at a major medical center in Cincinnati, Ohio. By the time Mom was evaluated by this physician, she was in moderate or mid-stage Alzheimer's disease (see Stages of Alzheimer's Disease in Chapter 3: Knowledge Is Power).

Being treated by this neurologist was exceptionally beneficial for Mom because he specialized in the care of Alzheimer's dementia. Her primary care physician could adequately care for her other health needs, but as Mom's dementia progressed, I sensed discomfort from her primary care physician in dealing with the dementia side of things. To say that the second neurologist was a godsend is putting it mildly. He took over management of Mom's dementia-related medications and offered suggestions for how to improve her quality of life and ease the increasing caregiving stress we were feeling. He valued what Mom had to say and conversed freely and easily with her. This physician cared for her until her transition into the nursing home. Since moving there, Mom has been managed primarily by a geriatric psychiatrist to address dementia-related medication management and a nurse practitioner to address her general health needs.

Conclusion

If you are a caregiver now or anticipate being one down the road, attend doctor visits as often as possible with your loved one, even if they are in the early stages of the disease. No one knows your loved one like you, the caregiver. The information you can share with the doctor is invaluable. And through this disease process, you will be called upon to act as advocate for your loved one as they are no longer able to advocate for themselves. The next chapter is aimed at helping you become an informed advocate for your loved one by educating yourself about Alzheimer's disease and preparing for what's to come.

Resources

Getting a Diagnosis

▶ The Alzheimer's Association 1–800–272–3900
Search this page for information on the steps to
diagnosis and the evaluation your loved one might
undergo during the medical work-up, as well as
guidance for finding the right doctor.
www.alz.org/alzheimers_disease_diagnosis.asp

▶ ADEAR (The Alzheimer's Disease Education
and Referral Center)
ADEAR provides information on the diagnostic
process when there is concern about changes in
memory and thinking. In addition, you will find
information on Alzheimer's disease basics as well as
information on causes, symptoms, and treatment.
www.nia.nih.gov/alzheimers

Finding a Geriatric Healthcare Professional

▶ The American Geriatrics Society (AGS)
Search at this link for a geriatric healthcare
professional. The physicians participating in this
referral service are members of the American
Geriatrics Society and are board certified in either
geriatrics or family practice. The family practice
physicians listed here have had additional training
to obtain a Certificate of Added Qualifications in
Geriatric Medicine.
www.healthinaging.org/find-a-geriatrics-healthcare-
professional/

Three

Knowledge Is Power

Even though my mother wasn't diagnosed with dementia of the Alzheimer's type until 2006, I began seeking information in 2003, as soon as she began the lengthy evaluation process to get to the bottom of her memory problems.

Educating myself on the premise that Mom might be diagnosed with Alzheimer's disease at some point could seem like putting the cart before the horse. But in my experience, it was empowering. The facts were that my mom's memory was declining, she was undergoing tests to determine the cause, and when she was diagnosed with mild cognitive impairment, I couldn't ignore her 60 percent chance of it someday progressing to Alzheimer's disease.

I've been attempting to educate myself on Alzheimer's disease for fourteen plus years now. In that time, I've seen a huge increase in both the amount of information available and ways to access that information. Educating yourself is one of the most effective things you can do as a caregiver to help your loved one.

An important first step is to become acquainted with the seven stages of Alzheimer's disease. While you might find reading about these stages depressing, it really does help to know what the future holds for both you and your loved one so you can be better prepared. Mom's decline was very slow, or so it seemed to my family and me. As Mom's memory declined and she progressed from a cognitive impairment to dementia, I would review these stages once or twice a year. It helped to clarify the changes I was seeing with Mom compared to the natural progression of the disease.

The Seven Stages of Alzheimer's Disease

Not everyone will experience the same symptoms or progress at the same rate. This seven-stage framework is based on a system developed by Barry Reisberg, MD, clinical director of the New York University School of Medicine's Silberstein Alzheimer's Institute.

Stage 1: No impairment (normal function): The person does not experience any memory problems. An interview with a medical professional does not show any evidence of symptoms of dementia.

Stage 2: Very mild cognitive decline (might be normal age-related changes or earliest signs of Alzheimer's disease): The person might feel as if he or she is having memory lapses—forgetting familiar words or the location of everyday objects. But no symptoms of dementia can be detected during a medical examination or by friends, family, or coworkers.

Stage 3: Mild cognitive decline (early-stage Alzheimer's disease can be diagnosed in some, but not all, individuals with these symptoms): Friends, family, or coworkers begin to notice difficulties. During a detailed medical interview, doctors might be able to detect problems in memory or concentration. Common stage 3 difficulties include:
- Noticeable problems coming up with the right word
- Trouble remembering names when introduced to new people

- Having noticeably greater difficulty performing tasks in social or work settings
- Forgetting material that one has just read
- Losing or misplacing a valuable object
- Increasing trouble with planning or organizing

Stage 4: Moderate cognitive decline (mild or early-stage Alzheimer's disease): At this point, a careful medical interview should be able to detect clear-cut symptoms in several areas:

- Forgetfulness of recent events
- Impaired ability to perform challenging mental arithmetic (for example, counting backward from 100 by 7s)
- Greater difficulty performing complex tasks, such as planning dinner for guests, paying bills, or managing finances
- Forgetfulness about one's own personal history
- Becoming moody or withdrawn, especially in socially or mentally challenging situations

Stage 5: Moderately severe cognitive decline (moderate or mid-stage Alzheimer's disease): Gaps in memory and thinking are noticeable, and individuals begin to need help with day-to-day activities. At this stage, those with Alzheimer's disease might:

- Be unable to recall their own address or telephone number or the high school or college from which they graduated
- Become confused about where they are or what day it is
- Have trouble with less challenging mental arithmetic (such as counting backward from 40 by subtracting 4s or from 20 by 2s)
- Need help choosing proper clothing for the season or the occasion

- Still remember significant details about themselves and their family
- Still require no assistance with eating or using the toilet

Stage 6: Severe cognitive decline (moderately severe or mid-stage Alzheimer's disease): Memory continues to worsen, personality changes might take place, and individuals need extensive help with daily activities. At this stage, individuals might:

- Lose awareness of recent experiences as well as of their surroundings
- Remember their own name but have difficulty with their personal history
- Distinguish familiar and unfamiliar faces but have trouble remembering the name of a spouse or caregiver
- Need help dressing properly and might, without supervision, make mistakes such as putting pajamas over daytime clothes or shoes on the wrong feet
- Experience major changes in sleep patterns such as sleeping during the day and becoming restless at night
- Need help handling details of toileting (for example, flushing the toilet, wiping, or disposing of tissue properly)
- Have increasingly frequent trouble controlling their bladder or bowels
- Experience major personality and behavioral changes, including suspiciousness and **delusions** (such as believing that their caregiver is an impostor) or compulsive, repetitive behavior like hand-wringing or tissue shredding
- Tend to wander or become lost

Stage 7: Very severe cognitive decline (Severe or late-stage Alzheimer's disease): In the final stage of this disease, individuals lose the ability to respond to their environment, to carry on a conversation and, eventually, to control movement. They might still say words or phrases. At this stage, individuals need help with much of their daily personal care, including eating or using the toilet. They might also lose the ability to smile, to sit without support and to hold their heads up. In addition, reflexes become abnormal, muscles grow rigid, swallowing becomes impaired.

Relatively speaking, your loved one will probably require less of your time and attention early in the disease process. This is the time to prepare for the future.

Getting Organized

As much as you can, prepare now by getting yourself organized as well as educated. Take advantage of the fact that your loved one will be better able to contribute to this process while they are less cognitively impaired.

Start by organizing your loved one's health history and include your loved one to fill in the blanks so that it's as thorough and accurate as possible. This can be as simple as creating a document that includes a list of illnesses and surgeries with their dates of occurrence, immunization record, allergies, date and result of most recent physical exam, test results, and eye- and dental-health records.

In addition to this basic information, you might consider starting a file that includes:

- An ongoing list of all physicians (past and present) with their contact information
- A separate, updated list of current physicians with their contact information
- Permission forms for providers to release your loved one's medical information to you or another designated family member

- An updated list of medications (prescription and over-the-counter)
- Pharmacy phone numbers
- Locations of important papers (see below)

Consider keeping electronic versions of these records in the cloud where other caregivers and family members can easily access information if they need to. Some cloud storage and sharing options like Google Drive also allow you to keep your loved one's calendar online where it is easy for everyone to access and update.

Advance Directives

If you haven't already done so, have a discussion about the importance of **advance directives** (a living will or durable power of attorney) with your loved one. As ADEAR explains, "Advance directives for healthcare are documents that communicate the healthcare wishes of a person. These decisions are then carried out after the person no longer can make decisions. In most cases, these documents must be prepared while the person is legally able to execute them."[1] Without these documents in place before a person reaches late-stage Alzheimer's disease, the caregiver is left to make decisions for a person who is likely unable to make their wishes known.

Procedures and interventions that should be addressed in advanced directives include:[2]

- Hospitalization including **DNH (do not hospitalize)**
- Careful hand feeding only
- Artificial nutrition and hydration-tube feeding
- **CPR (cardiopulmonary resuscitation)**
- **DNR (do not resuscitate)**
- Use of a ventilator
- Use of antibiotics
- Use of dialysis

- Treatment of pain
- Comfort and **palliative care**
- **Hospice care**

Other Important Documents

What additional information should a family caregiver organize? The answer to this question is different for every family. According to the Alzheimer's Disease Education and Referral Center (ADEAR), the following list is a great starting point as you're attempting to gather and organize your loved one's paperwork:

- Full legal name and residence
- Birth date and place and birth certificate
- Social Security and Medicare numbers
- Employer(s) and dates of employment
- Education and military records
- Sources of income and assets including investment income (stocks, bonds, property)
- Insurance policies, bank accounts, deeds, investments, and other valuables
- Most recent income tax return
- Money owed, to whom, and when payments are due
- Credit card account names and numbers
- Safe deposit box key and information
- Will and beneficiary information
- Durable power of attorney
- Living will and durable power of attorney for healthcare
- Where cash or other valuables might be kept in the home

I know this is a huge amount of information to gather, organize, and update. When viewed as a whole, this is a lot to accomplish and it might feel overwhelming. But if you break it down into several smaller steps, it will feel more manageable. For example, if you make it your goal to accomplish all of the items listed over the next year instead of next month, it's still a lot to accomplish but it becomes much more achievable.

Where to Get Information and Support

Below are some reliable resources for learning about various aspects of Alzheimer's disease that I found especially helpful early in the process.

Ten Real-Life Strategies for Dementia Caregiving

This list is a priceless resource from the Family Caregiver Alliance (www.caregiver.org/ten-real-life-strategies-dementia-caregiving). I discovered it after Mom moved to the nursing home, and wish I had known of its existence as we were caring for her at home. The ten strategies detailed are some of the most commonsense, user friendly, and invaluable pieces of advice on the subject of dementia caregiving I've found anywhere. If I could make it required reading, I would. It's that helpful!

The Alzheimer's Association

The Alzheimer's Association's (www.alz.org) mission is "[t]o eliminate Alzheimer's disease through the advancement of research; to provide and enhance care and support for all affected; and to reduce the risk of dementia through the promotion of brain health."[3]

Online resources: alz.org has a comprehensive publication library on a variety of Alzheimer's-related topics. All publications can be viewed, downloaded, and printed from your home computer. Print copies are available through your local Alzheimer's Association as well. In addition, because the internet has a vast amount of information, the Alzheimer's Association website became my fact-checker on numerous occasions.

Local chapters: The Alzheimer's Association chapter in your area will direct you to local educational offerings by the Alzheimer's Association. Over the years, I've attended many classes offered by the Alzheimer's Association. The topics ranged from caregiver workshops to the latest research trends. All have been worth my time. I also reached out to a contact at my local chapter. She became the person I contacted whenever I had a question that needed answering. It was invaluable to have access to a live person within the organization.

24/7 Helpline: Once I did need to use the 24/7 Helpline: 1–800–272–3900. An urgent question came up that could not wait for normal business hours. The man who assisted me was helpful, knowledgeable, competent, and caring.

Support groups: Alzheimer's Association sponsored support groups are places where you can exchange practical information on caregiving problems and possible solutions; talk through challenges and ways of coping; share feelings, needs, and concerns; and learn about resources available in your community. These support groups are led by a trained facilitator. Many offer supervised care for individuals with dementia during meeting times.

ADEAR (The Alzheimer's Disease Education and Referral Center)

ADEAR is the National Institute on Aging's Alzheimer's Disease Education and Referral Center. At their website (www.nia.nih.gov/alzheimers/about-adear-center) you will find current, comprehensive information and resources regarding Alzheimer's disease. The site has an Alzheimer's disease publications section. Many of these resources can be downloaded and printed from your home computer or ordered through ADEAR.

NIH Senior Health

This National Institutes of Health website (nihseniorhealth. gov) provides health and wellness information for older adults. The information on this site regarding Alzheimer's disease and caring for someone with Alzheimer's disease is more condensed than what you will find through the Alzheimer's Association or from ADEAR. However, the site provides excellent information.

Community Lectures

I attended lectures in my community given by physicians who were experts in the field of Alzheimer's disease. Most of these were provided by the Alzheimer's Association. I found others through local newspaper, radio, and TV ads. Others were put on by a long-term care facility in my area that caters exclusively to those with Alzheimer's disease. Lectures were positive experiences for a couple reasons. First, I was able to hear cutting-edge information from an expert in the field, which was always enlightening. Second, there was a feeling of kinship sitting among audience members who were all walking a similar road with their loved ones.

Updates in Drug Therapies

I tried to keep abreast of breakthroughs in Alzheimer's diease drug therapies. I did this because I continue to be interested in progress being made in Alzheimer's disease medications, but also because I wanted to know if there was anything on the horizon that might benefit Mom. There are many more drugs awaiting trials or in the middle of drug trials than are currently being used in the community. (See the Additional

Resources section at the end of this chapter for reputable information on current Alzheimer's-specific clinical trials.)

Support Groups

Support groups provide an opportunity to get out and meet others going through some of the same experiences. At a support group, you can share stories, get helpful hints for coping, and even obtain information about treatment options and long term care facilities. The Alzheimer's Association sponsors support groups in all fifty states. However, not everyone lives close to cities with Alzheimer's Association sponsored support groups. Local churches, senior centers, and your loved one's physician and office staff are good resources for information about caregiver support groups in your area.

Blogs and Online Message Boards

These resources are a way to receive many of the same benefits of a traditional support group whenever you're connected to the internet. However, before following any advice received from a blog or online message board, please consult with your loved one's physician to verify the safety and validity of the advice you've received.

Conclusion

In the next chapter, we'll explore strategies to enhance communication with your loved one as their abilities become increasingly impacted by Alzheimer's disease. This topic is essential because going forward you will notice that communicating well with your loved one plays a role in managing just about every caregiving challenge you will face.

Resources

General Information on Alzheimer's Disease and Caregiving

▶ **The Alzheimer's Association** 1–800–272–3900
This page provides an overview of Alzheimer's disease as well as links to other pages offering a wide variety of resources for caregivers and their families.
www.alz.org/alzheimers_disease_1973.asp

▶ **Family Caregiver Alliance**
Information on Alzheimer's disease, dementia, and mild cognitive impairment in a fact and tip sheet format. In addition, "Hands-on Skills for Caregivers" and "Pathways to Effective Communication for Healthcare Providers and Caregivers" are two publications that will be helpful at this stage of your journey.
www.caregiver.org/resources-health-issue-or-condition
www.caregiver.org/health-issues/dementia
www.caregiver.org/fact-sheets

▶ **Cleveland Clinic**
This glossary of terms provides you with an extensive list of pertinent terminology related to Alzheimer's disease.
my.clevelandclinic.org/health/articles/alzheimers-disease-glossary-of-terms

▶ **The Alzheimer's Project (video)**
HBO's The Alzheimer's Project presents a series of videos on many aspects of Alzheimer's disease of interest to family and caregivers.
www.hbo.com/alzheimers/index.html

▶ **The Forgetting: A Portrait of Alzheimer's (video)**
PBS's Emmy award-winning documentary based on the best-selling book by David Shenk.
www.pbs.org/program/forgetting/

Studies and Clinical Trials

▶ **ADEAR (The Alzheimer's Disease Education and Referral Center)**
Search for clinical trials and studies related to Alzheimer's disease, mild cognitive impairment, and caregiving.
www.nia.nih.gov/alzheimers/clinical-trials

Alzheimer's Disease Medications

▶ **National Institute on Aging**
A fact sheet detailing the current medications approved by the FDA to treat Alzheimer's disease, using understandable language for laypeople.
www.nia.nih.gov/alzheimers/publication/alzheimers-disease-medications-fact-sheet

Advance Planning

▶ **American Bar Association**
"Consumer's Toolkit for Health Care Advance Planning"
www.americanbar.org/groups/law_aging/resources/health_care_decision_making/consumer_s_toolkit_for_health_care_advance_planning.html

Resources for Young People

▶ **Books**
• *Striped Shirts and Flowered Pants: A Story about Alzheimer's Disease for Young Children* by Barbara Schnurbush (Magination Press, 2007)

- *Flowers for Grandpa Dan* by Connie McIntyre (Cache River Press, 2005)
- *What's Happening to Grandpa?* by Maria Shriver (Little, Brown Books for Young Readers, 2004)
- *Always My Grandpa: A story for Children about Alzheimer's Disease* by Linda Scacco (Magination Press, 2005)
- *The Graduation of Jake Moon* by Barbara Park (Alladin, 2002)

▶ **Videos**

If you have kids or teens who need help understanding what is happening to their family member, this page provides wonderful videos as well as literature (fact sheet printouts) to inform and educate young people on how Alzheimer's disease affects the brain. www.alz.org/living_with_alzheimers_just_for_kids_and_teens.asp

Four

Communication Strategies

Communication is at the heart of every relationship we have, whether we consider it to be effective or ineffective, positive or negative, or barely existent at all. When dementia starts to impact our loved one's ability to communicate, it accentuates just how important communication between people is. That's why I want to share a couple of experiences before I go any further. To give you some background, like so many mothers and daughters, Mom and I struggled intermittently with communication issues, especially throughout my teen and young adult years. And it's always made for a much more peaceful relationship with Mom to go along with her wishes. These long-practiced communication patterns—especially the second one—have continued, at least in part, throughout much of her disease. As you read this book, you might notice that my family and I skirted around certain issues instead of facing them head on, and I'm sure we're not alone. It can feel like a juggling act to make the ongoing adjustments necessary to promote effective communication with our loved ones as the disease progresses while still being influenced by those old patterns.

New Communication Techniques

Of all the challenges Alzheimer's disease poses to caregivers, none is so frustrating to manage on a practical level or so devastating to accept on an interpersonal level as what Alzheimer's disease does to communication. How then do you communicate with a person whose ability has been diminished by dementia? Well, if you're willing to learn some communication techniques that might feel uncomfortable and unnatural at first, you'll be taking a giant step in the right direction. Keep in mind that becoming comfortable with this new way of communicating with your loved one takes time and practice. Also, there's no one formula for effective communication with people with dementia. You'll need to figure out what works best for both of you while acknowledging that, as the disease progresses, you might need to adopt different techniques. At times, this can feel as uncomfortable as learning a new language. Acknowledge when something doesn't work and try a different technique the next time. Forgive yourself for making mistakes. Just keep trying!

One thing I can tell you from my experience is that being able to effectively communicate with your loved one (even some of the time) can make your role as caregiver more rewarding and less stressful.

Below are some suggestions I've come up with that can ease communication with your loved one:

- **Always call your loved one by name.** For those with dementia, their name is a recognizable word attached to them (usually from birth). Calling them by name helps to get their attention.
- **Use familiar words, names, and phrases.** In Mom's presence, I now refer to my dad as Tom because if I call him Dad, Mom thinks I'm referring to her dad. If your loved one always referred to soft drinks as *soda,*

continue to do so. In other words, it doesn't matter how common a term, word, or name is if it's not the term, word, or name your loved one used. Stick to what your loved one is familiar with.

- **Try distraction if communication breaks down.** If you're attempting to assist your loved one in getting dressed and they are uncooperative, try to distract them with something else for a few minutes and then retry the original task. For example, have a basket of clean laundry handy for your loved one to help you fold.
- **Limit distractions.** While distraction can work when you do it intentionally, limit outside distractions when you're trying to get your loved one's attention or trying to get them to do something. The less stimuli they have to deal with, the better chance your message will be received. The sights and sounds coming from TVs, radios, and computers can be very distracting. Try turning them off if you're having trouble getting your loved one's attention.

Body Language and Touch

Communication involves more than simply talking with another person. We communicate most certainly with words, but also with facial expressions, eye contact, body language, and touch. We can encourage, support, and reassure with our words. But our facial expressions can communicate patience, care, and concern as well. Maintaining eye contact during communication can show someone that you value what they are saying and also aid in keeping their attention. Our body language can impart an attitude of patience and care. Finally, touch: through touch we can convey safety, respect, and love.

I'd like to share an interaction that I observed between a resident and one of the nurses at Mom's dementia unit. From what I could tell, this resident didn't seem to be in pain. She had just eaten dinner, so hunger was probably not the issue. But by the way she was behaving, something was clearly wrong—she was very agitated and vocalizing loudly. During our afterdinner walk, Mom and I passed her several times as she sat in the hall just outside the dining room. All of a sudden, I noticed that things had quieted down considerably. I looked in the woman's direction and saw the nurse standing next to her, slowly combing her fingers through the woman's hair. The woman's eyes were closed and she had the most blissful expression on her face. I looked at the nurse and smiled. She simply said: "She loves this." Maybe the woman's family had told the nurse how much she loved having her hair stroked, or maybe the nurse discovered it in the course of providing care to her over time. Whatever the reason, a soothing touch by a caring and thoughtful caregiver was the remedy for her discomfort.

When interacting with your loved one, convey an unhurried, easygoing attitude. You have a better chance of positively influencing the mood and tone of your loved one if you approach them with a relaxed attitude. In addition to maintaining eye contact, smile and appear interested in what your loved one has to say, even if you don't understand them. You don't need to have dementia to appreciate someone being interested in what you say or do. This caring act sends your loved one a message of your approval.

The way you walk into a room or how you approach and greet your loved one can affect their mood and behavior. When approaching your loved one, do so from the front. Allow them to see you before they hear you. Your face might be more recognizable than just your voice, and recognition is reassuring. If you reach out to touch your loved one, also do so from the front to avoid startling them. Avoid sudden movements that could be perceived as threatening. Be aware of how close you can be to your loved one before they show signs of feeling threatened, overwhelmed, or uncomfortable and then adjust your stance accordingly. You can still show your love and affection while respecting your loved one's personal space. Offer a hand to hold instead.

Keeping It Simple

Keeping sentences and phrases simple has been a particular challenge for me. It's just not the way I normally talk. And even though I've had years to practice and improve upon this skill, it still requires a conscious effort to simplify my communication with Mom. Below are some pointers I learned that might help you:

- **Speak clearly using short, concise words and sentences.** Directions that might seem straightforward and easily understood by you and me can (and should) be simplified to make them more easily understood by your loved one.

Instead of:	Say this:
"Let's go to the bathroom to wash our hands because it's time to get ready for dinner."	"Let's wash our hands." (Demonstrate to orient your loved one to the task if needed.) After hands are washed, say: "Let's eat dinner."

- **Ask questions that could be answered with yes, no, or a few words.** The same reason you use simple and concise wording when offering directions and explanations applies when asking a question.

Instead of:	Say this:
"Do you want gravy on your mashed potatoes and roast beef, and butter on your bread?	Show your loved one the gravy and ask: "Would you like gravy on your mashed potatoes?" After they have answered that question, do the same with the roast beef and bread. Ask: "Do you want gravy on your roast beef?" Then: "Do you want butter on your bread?" Showing your loved one the bread and butter, or demonstrating putting butter on bread might be helpful

- **Use concrete words.**

Instead of:	Say this:
"Let's get going."	"Let's go to the store."

- **Use written reminders if they're helpful.** Simple written reminders might work if your loved one is able to read and understand written words. For example, a sign at the bathroom sink could read: "Wash hands then turn off water." Or a sign on the inside of the front door could read: "After you close the door, lock it." Or a sign on the milk jug could read: "Put milk back in refrigerator."

Slowing Down

Slowing down is a particular challenge given the speed at which we live our lives. Even if your loved one was the type of person who multitasked with ease or moved through life at 100 miles per hour, the effects of dementia will change that capability over time. You might not even be aware of how fast you talk or how intricate and complex your speech is until your loved one starts having difficulty understanding you. My advice is to slow down. Slow *way* down and avoid acting rushed. Imagine watching the credits roll at the end of a television program. They are rolling so fast that you can't read them all, much less comprehend them before they're off the screen and a new list appears. What if you were quizzed on what you just saw? Could you pass? Maybe, if they were shown to you more slowly.

Below are some suggestions for slowing down:
- **Show patience.** It has a calming effect.
- **Talk slowly and clearly.** It might be easier for your loved one to differentiate words if each word is spoken separately and distinctly. This takes practice.
- **Repeat yourself** if your loved one does not respond to your question or statement, but first give them time to respond.

- **Don't interrupt.** Clearminded people can lose their train of thought if interrupted. Imagine what it must feel like if it's a struggle to express the simplest thought. Get in the habit of responding only when your loved one has finished speaking.
- **Take deep breaths** periodically to remind yourself to slow down.

Tone of Voice

It's amazing to me how reactive Mom is to tone of voice, even now. To illustrate, I visit her at the nursing home twice per week during mealtimes. After a difficult month of feeding her, I had reached my limit after she threw her buttered bread with enough gusto to send a glass of milk flying. As I was cleaning up the splattered milk, I expressed my frustration by saying, "I don't know how Dad does this every day. Mom you're really making it hard on me right now." Mom responded in kind, matching my frustration with indignation. Sounding irritated by my scolding, she raised her voice and expressed her displeasure by stringing together a group of *words* that were completely unintelligible to me. You might think after all these years of practice I would have mastered communication with my mom. I felt guilty for losing my patience with her but, at the same time, I was aware that I had an increasing feeling of dread every time I entered Mom's unit for a visit. I recognized that my being shorttempered with Mom during our visits was not in her best interest, and my feeling irritable and reactive whenever Mom behaved like a person with dementia wasn't good for either of us. I decided to limit my visits to once a week for a while. Doing so gave me a chance to recharge so I could visit Mom with a refreshed attitude.

Below are some suggestions for managing tone of voice:

- **Stay positive.** Messages are generally better received if delivered with a positive tone.
- **Adopt a tone of empathy.** For example, if your loved one is having a hard time expressing themself verbally, you could say: "Sometimes it's hard to get the right words out, isn't it?"
- **Avoid questions like,** "Do you remember . . . ?" Your loved one might view this as a test. This might remind your loved one of what they no longer know or remember, and might provoke anxiety and agitation.
- **Offer thanks and praise** for their efforts. It doesn't matter how well the job was done or even what the task was, for that matter. They'll just feel good being recognized for the effort.

Repetition

Early in the disease process your loved one might repeat things like a broken record. This is very common. For the first few years, Mom did in fact repeat herself like a broken record. Below is a typical conversation I'd have with Mom as her disease progressed:

Mom: Are you dating anyone?

Me: Yes.

Mom: Who?

Me: Paul.

Mom: Paul who?

Me: Paul Neuzil.

Mom: Oh! . . . Well, dinner was lovely, honey. Are you dating anyone?

I wouldn't offer more information because Mom didn't ask for any other details. At this point, when Mom saw Paul, she knew his name. And when Paul and I were together, she seemed to know that we were married.

For a few years, this conversation took place every time my Mom and I talked, either in person or on the phone. And it was repeated over and over and *over!* Could I have answered any differently to calm the situation, to orient Mom to the fact that Paul and I were married, or to stop the line of questioning permanently? I doubt it because there was no situation to calm. Mom was perfectly content with my answer. I didn't want to risk upsetting her by reminding her that she might have forgotten something, and she seemed to need to ask that question almost like a conversation starter.

A few years later, the devastating toll Alzheimer's disease takes on memories was even more apparent. To illustrate:

Mom: Are you dating anyone?
Me: Yes.
Mom: Who?
Me: Paul.
Mom: Paul who?
Me: Paul Neuzil.
Mom: Oh! Do you think you two might ever get married?
Me: Mom, we're married.
Mom: WHAT?!!!
Me: You know that, Mom. We've been married for a long time.
Mom: I don't believe it! Why didn't anyone tell me? TOM, DID YOU KNOW AMY AND PAUL GOT MARRIED?!!! WHY DIDN'T YOU TELL ME?!!!

Because this occurred in a public setting and was causing a scene, I insisted Dad leave immediately with Mom. I simply didn't know what to do. I watched my parents walk to the car with Mom giving Dad a tonguelashing the entire way. What could I have done differently? Everything!

I can't tell you that I never made that kind of mistake again. But I can tell you that that incident was the catalyst to make some changes in the way I communicated with my mother. It took time and it took practice.

While the previous example was horrendous, this next one showed signs of improvement:

Mom: Are you and Paul married?

Me: Yes, we are.

Mom: What? Why didn't you tell me?

Me: I'm so sorry Mom. I thought I told you.

Mom: That's OK, but I wish I could have been there.

Me: I wish you could have been there too.

Was it 100 percent truthful? Does it have to be? Or possibly, and most importantly, as I learned through trial and error, is there any earthly reason I need to remind Mom of something she doesn't remember anymore?

Embarrassing Situations

People with Alzheimer's disease often do not have the same social restraints others have and might do or say things we find embarrassing. Mom's dementia doctor demonstrated a great (and humorous) way to handle situations that are uncomfortable to us as caregivers.

At a routine visit with Mom's dementia neurologist, my sister Mary and I were sharing some information with him. I think Mom wanted to contribute something to the conversation, so she lifted up her shirt to expose her belly and began lightly and rhythmically beating it like a tomtom. When she finished, she looked at us and said, "What do you think of that?" While Mary and I exchanged uncomfortable glances, her doctor smiled and exclaimed: "Dolores, that is the first drum solo anyone has done in this room today! Thank you!" Mom was elated. I've never forgotten the expression on her face or the gratitude I felt for this sensitive doctor for responding the way he did. He made Mom feel appreciated. This doctor's simple statement demonstrated to us the benefits of positive communication even when we, as caregivers, are uncomfortable with things our loved ones say or do.

Nonverbal Clues

As Mom has entered the late stages of Alzheimer's disease, I've become increasingly dependent on her nonverbal cues when trying to decipher what she's attempting to convey. Her verbal skills have declined to a level that makes it almost impossible to understand anything she says. However, she was always a very expressive person when she talked, and her facial expressions and body language were as much a part of how she communicated as the words she used. Gratefully those traits have largely remained intact. For example, if Mom is not pleased with her meal, she doesn't have the words to say she doesn't like it or doesn't want to eat it. Instead, she gets her point across by looking at me, rolling her eyes, and raising one side of her upper lip in disgust. Point taken.

When I visit her and find her restless, irritable, or agitated, I often can't tell the reason for her bad mood. But if I approach her with a empathetic tone, hoping to convey that I care about her discomfort whether I can make it better for her or not, she responds much more positively. Phrases like "I'm sorry you're having a hard time today, Mom" have helped me out of many a jam.

Through the process of trying to understand Mom's nonverbal or hard-to-understand communications, my family and I discovered something that I wish we had known sooner. When you're having trouble deciphering what your loved one is trying to communicate, scan the scene for clues. It takes practice to be able to take in the surroundings while listening to your loved one, who might be making little to no sense with their words. But it really does help make sense of things when their words don't. For example, when Mom is irritable, she doesn't have the ability to explain what's bothering her. Sometimes we can intervene and improve her mood by changing her environment, especially if it's loud and chaotic. But if that doesn't change her mood for the better, we start looking for other things that could be contributing to her irritability or discomfort. Is she hungry? Do her clothes or undergarments need changing? Is she in pain? Sometimes we're able to pinpoint the irritant, intervene, and eliminate it. However, there are times we simply cannot decipher the cause or we can't do anything to remedy it. It's possible that Mom is irritable just because of the effects of Alzheimer's disease. In those instances, we do our best to be a calm and supportive presence for her.

Visiting a Person with Alzheimer's Disease[1]

Visitors are important to people with Alzheimer's disease. They might not always remember who their visitors are, but the human connection has value. Here are some ideas to share with someone who is planning to visit a person with the disease.

- Plan the visit for the time of day when the person with Alzheimer's disease is at their best.
- Consider bringing along an activity, such as something familiar to read or photo albums to look at, but be prepared to skip it if necessary.
- Be calm and quiet. Avoid using a loud tone of voice or talking to the person as if he or she were a child.

- Respect the person's personal space and don't get too close.
- Try to establish eye contact and call the person by name to get his or her attention.
- Remind the person who you are if he or she doesn't seem to recognize you.
- Don't argue if the person is confused. Respond to the feelings you hear being communicated, and distract the person to a different topic if necessary.
- Remember not to take it personally if the person doesn't recognize you, is unkind, or responds angrily. He or she is reacting out of confusion.

Conclusion

I don't mean to minimize the communication challenges we all face as caregivers or to oversimplify the solutions to combat them. But the techniques illustrated throughout this chapter *usually* work for us. When you begin experimenting with techniques to communicate more effectively with your loved one, consider their point of view. Remember that the effects of dementia alter their reality. Through trial and error, I've learned that the communication between us goes much more smoothly when I try to live in Mom's world with her.

This last example happens regularly during my visits with Mom in the nursing home. I used to find her walking the halls of her dementia unit until she took a couple of falls, and both my family and the staff at the nursing home decided that Mom would be safer if she spent her waking hours in a wheelchair unless someone was available to walk with her. Now, nine times out of ten, I find her roaming the halls in her wheelchair. Movement is soothing to her. If she's coming toward me, I wait until she sees me before I say anything to her. If she's not, I catch up to her until she sees me and say, "Hi Mom." Before her language skills declined so much, she'd usually smile and say something like, "Hi. What did you get here?" I believe that sentence to be a combination of "What are you doing here?" and "How did you get here?" (But really, who knows?) Now, she'll say something using sounds in the place of words. "I wanted to see you." I say. Sometimes Mom is OK with a hug, but not always. Then I push her back to her room to drop off her wheelchair. I reach out both hands and ask her if she'd like to take a walk. She reaches out to me, grabs my hands and stands, and then we walk together.

Resources

Help with Communication Issues

▶ The Alzheimer's Association 1–800–272–3900
Help for addressing communication challenges
including tips to help the person with Alzheimer's
disease communicate.
www.alz.org/care/dementia-communication-tips.asp

▶ ADEAR (The Alzheimer's Disease Education
and Referral Center)
Several publications listed on this page address
communication and Alzheimer's disease. All can be
downloaded or ordered in hard copy.
www.nia.nih.gov/alzheimers/topics/caregiving

▶ Family Caregiver Alliance
"Guidelines for Better Communication" is a
publication to assist you with communication
challenges between you and your loved one.
www.caregiver.org/guidelines-better-communication-
brain-impaired-adults

▶ Books
*I was Thinking: Unlocking the Door to Successful
Conversations with Loved Ones with Cognitive Loss* by
Diana Waugh RN BSN (Lulu.com, 2008)

I received this book from a friend soon after my
mother was diagnosed with Alzheimer's disease.
This book was an invaluable resource when I was
struggling to communicate with her. It is filled with
real-life examples that I was able to incorporate into
actual conversations with my mom.

▶ **Videos**

The Alzheimer's Project
www.hbo.com/alzheimers/index.html

Five

Help with Hygiene

When Mom was diagnosed with mild cognitive impairment in 2003, the main issue we were aware of was loss of her short-term memory. But within a few years, her cognitive abilities declined so much that her diagnosis was changed to dementia of the Alzheimer's type. She was having more and more difficulty with complex tasks, such as planning and preparing meals, holiday preparations, and balancing the checkbook. However, it was hygiene that became the single most problematic, ongoing issue we faced regarding Mom's care.

Previously, Mom had been able to tend to her hygiene needs independently. She had always been conscientious regarding her appearance and all hygiene-related issues, so when we started noticing a decline in her appearance and hygiene, we became very concerned. We looked for ways to handle this delicate matter in the most respectful and least offensive manner possible.

The reason this issue was so challenging for us (as it is for most caregivers) is because it's such a personal and private subject. Our family wanted to be sensitive to Mom's feelings, considerate of her dignity, and mindful of her self-respect. But how do you accomplish all of that when your loved one is unaware that a problem exists and believes that they are taking care of their hygiene just fine?

We struggled mightily with this dilemma. We struggled to find the right approach with Mom. We struggled to choose the right words to discuss her hygiene issues with her. And we tried different tactics in the hope of finding some that worked. For example, Dad joined Mom in the shower to assist her and offer her direction as needed. When he couldn't do that, we encouraged her to take a bath rather than a shower. We figured it would be easier logistically to help her if she was taking a bath instead. Before bedtime, Dad would lay out Mom's clothes for the next day in the order she was to dress herself (i.e., underwear first, shoes last).

In addition, we put simple checklists in the bathroom labeled *Morning* and *Evening*. They looked something like this:

Morning	Evening
Use toilet	Take a shower or bath
Take off pajamas	Put on pajamas
Put on deodorant	Brush teeth
Put on clean clothes	Use toilet
Brush teeth	
Comb hair	

Mom was able to read, but her comprehension was becoming questionable at times. So Dad explained the need for the checklists to her by saying: "We're both getting older. This is to make sure we're getting all of our self-care done."

Bathing and Showering

Bathing issues became some of our biggest challenges. Bathing became a topic that often provoked anger in Mom. Truthfully, we handled her resistance to assistance with bathing by and large by acquiescing to her wishes. Occasionally she had days when she seemed more like her old self and less resistant about help with showering and hygiene. Unfortunately, nothing we tried was successful for any length of time, and hygiene continued to be a struggle.

Here's a painful example. Because Mom had primarily taken a shower in the evening throughout her adult life, it made sense to keep shower or bath time in the evening. Sometimes, however, depending on Mom's schedule for the day, it was more convenient to have her shower in the morning. But if she got up and dressed before Dad noticed, it was all but impossible to get her to agree to take a shower. In her mind, she must have taken one already because she was dressed.

One rare morning when I was able to coax her to take a shower, I stayed within earshot in case she called out for help or needed something. I was fairly certain that she was unable to shower by herself, but I decided to peek in the shower to confirm what I believed to be true. I found Mom cowering in the corner, staring at the water coming out of the showerhead. My heart sank. I hated that it took witnessing my mother in such a vulnerable and frightened position to force a change in the way we were managing this troublesome issue. I made a promise at that moment that I would never put her through that again.

Later that day I spoke with my sister Mary. We discussed alternative bathing methods. Sponge bathing came up as a possibility, but we questioned the logistics of having to rinse off the soap outside a tub or shower. After some research into rinse-free bathing products, we found one worth trying.

I want to share with you the other changes we made because they worked amazingly well for us. I share them, too, because we struggled for a long time and experimented with many different things before we stumbled on ones that worked with Mom. I'm not saying that our methods are ideal and are the way you should handle hygiene issues with your loved one. (Where good hygiene is concerned, I've come to believe that when you find a way that works for you, that's about ideal as it gets.) But, using the system we came up with, Mary successfully bathed Mom twice a week for over two years.

Below are some of Mary's hygiene solutions that worked well for us, as well as suggestions from professional organizations that deal with issues related to Alzheimer's disease. The Alzheimer's Association and ADEAR are both good resources for information on how to handle hygiene with your loved one.

Preparation

Being prepared ahead of time will simplify the bathing process for both you and your loved one, so have all supplies readily available before you start:

- Soap or rinse-free body wash
- Shampoo and conditioner or rinse-free shampoo (rinse-free shampoo is drying to the scalp, so we limited it to one time per week)
- Moisturizing lotion for skin
- Deodorant
- Towels and washcloths
- Robe or clean clothing

It also helps to have plenty of washcloths soaking in the bath water. If one becomes soiled, pitch it and reach for a clean one. This saves time and prevents contamination of the clean bath water.

Comfort and Safety while Bathing

- Make sure the room and water temperature are comfortable for your loved one
- Have warm soapy water ready in the sink or a basin if you plan to give a sponge bath
- Have an absorbent towel on the toilet lid so your loved one is not sitting on a hard surface

We'll cover safety in detail in Chapter 6: Safety First, but a few details are important to talk about here. Many accidents happen during bath and shower time regardless of one's age or health status. Taking some safety precautions can help ensure your loved one's safety during bath time:

- Install non-skid strips on slippery tub and shower floors
- Have handrails installed in the bath and shower
- Consider getting a handheld showerhead so your loved one can sit in the tub while bathing; a handheld showerhead also makes it easy to spray only those areas that need washing while reducing difficulty for caregivers assisting in bathing
- Make sure the bathroom door has a knob that can't be locked from the inside so your loved one can't lock themselves in when using the bathroom
- *Never* leave your loved one alone in the bath or shower

Once all the preparations are made, it can sometimes be exceedingly challenging to get your loved one to actually take a bath or shower. It certainly was for us! Below are some of Mary's successful tactics for convincing Mom to bathe.

Diversion

The words *bath* and *shower* were agitating to Mom. Instead, Mary would say, "Let's get cleaned up" or "I'll help you smell good." Both to get Mom into the bathroom and to keep her engaged and cooperative during the bath, Mary sang familiar songs and told familiar stories. If Mom couldn't be coaxed into the bathroom with songs or stories, Mary would try other diversions such as, "Let me show you something" or "Smell this new lotion" or "Look at these new towels."

Once Mary started with the bath or shower, she kept the process moving along quickly as Mom's attention span and tolerance for a bath lasted only a short while. Mary also encouraged her to participate as much as she was able. Another challenge was that Mom became very anxious when she was completely undressed. So Mary only uncovered or undressed the body part she was bathing, and then immediately covered that area up with clothing or a large towel before going on to the next area.

Timing and Flexibility

If your loved one always bathed at a specific time of day, try to keep bathing at that same time. If not, try to establish a bathing routine as early as possible, choosing a time when they're the most calm and agreeable and when you feel calm and not rushed.

Mary allowed plenty of time for Mom's bath. If she had time constraints, she didn't initiate the bath. Mary also planned ahead for special occasions and holidays. Planning the bath a day or two before a holiday allowed for some flexibility if Mom was uncooperative the first time. I think Mary's attitude was one of the reasons she was so successful at bathing Mom: she was able to bring a time-is-not-an-issue attitude to a task that could be stress producing for both of them.

Bathing can be scary and uncomfortable for some people with Alzheimer's disease. Being gentle and respectful and patient and calm can work wonders. If your loved one still refuses to take a bath or shower, try a sponge bath. If they are having a bad day and behave as if a full sponge bath might be too much to cope with, limit it to the *essentials* (perineal area, armpits, hands, and face).

If all efforts fail, shower aides (nurse aides) can be hired to give your loved one their showers. Your loved one might cooperate better with a healthcare professional than with a close family member or friend.

Grooming

Grooming is often one of the first signs that your loved one could be struggling to care for themselves. A scruffy beard on a man who was always clean shaven or a woman who's stopped wearing makeup or starts applying it inappropriately are red flags that should not be ignored. In Mom's case, she simply stopped wearing makeup. Timewise, this change corresponded to the beginning of Mom's struggles with hygiene.

In general, encourage your loved one to maintain the grooming routines they've always followed. If your loved one has always used makeup, encourage her to do so and assist as needed. (To avoid eye injuries, it's best that she not apply eye makeup herself.) And if your loved one wants to shave, have him use an electric razor.

Where your loved one can't maintain their routine, make adaptations where you need to. Mary dried and styled Mom's hair when she would tolerate it. If not, Mom's hair would air dry. We also occasionally took Mom to the hair stylist to have her hair washed with traditional shampoo, cut, and styled. However, some barbers and hairstylists will come to your home if that is more convenient for you and your loved one.

Because your loved one could scratch themself or others, it's also important to keep your loved one's nails clean and trimmed. Toenails also need to be trimmed. If Mom would tolerate it, Mary would soak Mom's feet in a basin of warm water and trim her nails while she was talking with Dad or watching TV.

Dressing

Getting your loved one dressed, whether or not they've bathed, is another important and potentially problematic aspect of personal hygiene. Dementia caregiving experts stress the need to limit the decisions involved in dressing for your loved one. They also recommend storing out-of-season clothing away from clothing routinely worn until it is needed.

Fortunately, depending on the season, Mom loved to wear khakis and a white T-shirt or turtleneck. We filled her drawers with those items, as we knew that would most likely be a pleasing choice for her. This tactic really simplified things for us and the change was not at all difficult to implement. As Mom's dementia progressed, we simplified her shoe choices too. Shoes with elevated heels were replaced with sturdy walking shoes with non-skid soles.

Mom routinely dressed herself in the morning. As she became more cognitively impaired, the final product wasn't always ... appropriate. For example, if Mom dressed before we could offer guidance, she might put her clothes on over her pajamas. However, in the scheme of things, I never really considered that to be a big deal. But if Mom insisted on sleeping in her clothes, it became a bigger deal because, upon waking the next morning she would get dressed for the day, adding another layer of clothing to what she was already wearing. Trying to convince Mom that she was wearing three layers made for an exercise in futility and frustration.

To better understand the difficulties people with Alzheimer's disease have when dressing themselves, try to put yourself in their shoes (pun intended). Pay attention to the number of steps it takes to dress yourself, taking into account the outside temperature and weather, dressing appropriately for the day's activities, putting undergarments and clothing on in the correct order, etc. Then imagine accomplishing all that if you had dementia. Dressing is a complex process. Whether your loved one requires little assistance or considerably more, acknowledge their effort with gratitude and praise. It truly is an accomplishment.

Oral Hygiene

Have you ever heard someone say that the mouth is one of the most germ-laden parts of our bodies? Research has actually been done on the relationship between periodontal disease, tooth loss, and infection. Periodontal disease has been shown to be a cause of bacterial and aspiration pneumonia[1] (see Chapter 10: The Final Chapter). In other words, good oral care has been proven effective in decreasing the incidence of not only tooth loss but also **pneumonia**. Isn't that a powerful incentive to tend to your loved one's teeth and gums (or dentures if they've already lost their teeth)? If only it were that easy.

For several years, Mom was able to brush her teeth with verbal instructions from one of us. But as her disease progressed, she required someone else to brush them for her, and she doesn't like that one bit. The best way we've found to handle Mom's resistance is to use a foam-tipped applicator dipped in diluted mouthwash.

In addition, it might help if you brush your teeth at the same time to demonstrate how it's done. Make sure your instructions are simple and straightforward (see Chapter 4: Communication Strategies), giving one instruction at a time. As with all other aspects of hygiene and personal grooming, allow your loved one to do as much for themselves as possible for as long as they are able. And be sure to praise them afterwards. If you do need to brush your loved one's teeth, try a long-handled, angled, or electric toothbrush. It might be easier to manage than a traditional one. If they have dentures, those need to be cleaned daily, and you might need to help with this as well.

Which brings me to the best piece of advice suited for almost any caregiving challenge: if your loved is having trouble doing something or outright refuses, try again later. (Obviously, this does not apply to issues where their safety is at risk.)

Approaching a task from another angle might be as simple as wording your request differently or using a different tone of voice (see Chapter 4: Communication Strategies), looking for a change in your loved one's mood, or taking advantage of another opportunity. For example, if you're already helping your loved one in the bathroom, you might suggest that they also brush their teeth. And vice versa; if they're in the bathroom brushing their teeth, you might suggest that they use the toilet.

In addition to daily oral care, be sure to take your loved one for routine dental checkups as often as their dentist recommends. Some dentists specialize in treating those with Alzheimer's disease, and you might find it helpful to seek out one who does, both to facilitate your loved one's care and for the additional support a specialist can provide to you.

Toileting and Incontinence

Without question, this is the most difficult topic for me to discuss as it pertains to my mom. Maybe if my family and I had been successful in managing this issue, I would feel more comfortable discussing it. I could then share what worked for us in the hope that you could be helped in your situation. The truth is, we struggled to manage this challenging issue at home. And it really didn't get managed well until Mom moved to the nursing home. However, there is a lot of good information available on this subject to help caregivers and their loved ones.

To begin with, issues with incontinence usually begin in the later stages of Alzheimer's disease. Bowel incontinence and bladder incontinence are separate issues and one might occur without the other. If your loved one starts having problems with incontinence, have their physician perform a thorough evaluation to rule out other causes (such as urinary tract infection, uncontrolled diabetes, or enlarged prostate) before assuming it's dementia related. Sudden changes in temperament or behavior are often an indicator of illness in those with dementia and should not be ignored.

Steps for Managing Incontinence

If the underlying cause is determined to be dementia related, there are steps you can take to manage the incontinence:

- If your loved one is able to move about independently, leave the bathroom door open so the toilet is visible
- Try putting a relevant picture or sign on the bathroom door to cue your loved one to its location
- Get in the habit of encouraging a bathroom visit after meals and every two to three hours during waking hours
- Learn the cues that indicate your loved one needs to use the bathroom (these might include fidgeting, restlessness, irritability, or pulling at clothes), and respond quickly
- Provide your loved one with clothes that are simple to remove (for example, pants with an elastic waistband are just so much easier and faster to remove than those with buttons, hooks, and zippers)
- As much as possible, honor your loved one's need for privacy during bathroom time
- Be as prepared as possible (locate bathrooms and have an extra set of clothes, disposable briefs, incontinence pad, or adult diaper and disposable wipes with you in case of an accident)

All of that being said, even if you're the most diligent and prepared caregiver, accidents will occur from time to time. Accidents are hard on everyone. Even though your loved one is cognitively impaired, society tells us that having an accident is embarrassing or shameful when we're adults. Stay calm, reassure your loved one, and be understanding.

Alternatives to Underwear

If your loved one's incontinence gets to a point that you're considering alternatives to underwear, you have a few choices. There are pluses and minuses to all three. Ultimately, you will have to evaluate your loved one's needs and choose based on your individual situation.

- **Incontinence pads** fit directly into regular underwear. The upside is that your loved one continues to wear the underwear they are used to. The downside is that the pads need to be changed about as often as your loved one regularly goes to the bathroom.
- **Disposable briefs** are worn like underwear, which is a plus if your loved one needs more protection than an incontinence pad can offer and they are concerned about the aesthetics of an adult diaper. The disadvantage of disposable briefs is that, in order to change them, clothing from the waist down needs to be removed.
- **Adult diapers** fasten on at the side like a baby diaper does. Changing adult diapers requires only that clothing be pulled down, not completely removed. That is a plus. However, despite being cognitively impaired, your loved one might attach a stigma to wearing adult diapers.

Conclusion

If you've tried everything and you're still meeting resistance with bathing, grooming, dressing, oral hygiene, or toileting or incontinence issues, bring it to the attention of your loved one's physician. In addition, contact the Alzheimer's Association for support, guidance, and a fresh perspective.

Resources

Help with Hygiene Issues

▶ **The Alzheimer's Association** 1–800–272–3900
Incontinence and toileting, bathing, dressing and
grooming, and dental care are discussed in detail.
www.alz.org/care/alzheimers-dementia-daily-plan.asp

▶ **ADEAR** (The Alzheimer's Disease Education
and Referral Center)
Several publications, addressing all aspects of hygiene,
are available to order or download and copy at home.
www.nia.nih.gov/alzheimers/topics/caregiving—
everyday

▶ **Family Caregiver Alliance**
Dementia-specific publications on all aspects of
hygiene and "Assistive Technology" are helpful guides
when you face hygiene challenges with your loved
one.
www.caregiver.org/fact-sheets

▶ **Videos**
Peter Rabins Alzheimer's Family Support Center:
"Dressing and Bathing—Memory and Alzheimer's
Disease."
www.youtube.com/watch?v=iLU_
foo1c4I&feature=youtu.be

Six

Safety First

Of all the issues caregivers face, their loved one's safety, both inside and outside the home, is among the most challenging and important. While all elderly people are at high risk for injuries from accidents, the chances that a person with Alzheimer's disease will experience a serious injury from a fall or other accident are considerably greater. In the previous chapter on hygiene, I touched on some of the safety issues related to bathing and showering. These included dealing with slippery bathroom floors, tubs, and showers; having doorknobs that can't be locked from inside the bathroom; and never leaving your loved one alone in a bath or shower. In this chapter, I'll address safety issues more generally.

As I began researching safety, I was reminded again how Alzheimer's disease affects people at different speeds and presents them with different challenges. Because each situation is different and safety issues can change as the disease progresses, it's important to evaluate your loved one's safety needs on a regular basis. At different stages of Mom's disease, we had to address a variety of safety issues; her behaviors and limitations necessitated careful monitoring and occasional intervention on our part. Initially, those issues focused primarily on driving and in-home safety, especially fall prevention.

Falling

The bathroom isn't the only place where your loved one can slip, trip, and fall. Falling became an issue as Mom's dementia progressed. When she walked, she no longer noticed what was in her path, especially if an object was close to or on the ground. This often caused her to bump herself, trip, and even fall. For example, there were a couple of areas in the wall-to-wall carpet in her house that had begun to pull away from the floor, causing ripples in the carpet. They weren't large areas, but given the fact that Mom didn't notice what was at floor level, she began tripping on the ripples. After weighing our options (either replacing the carpet or having it stretched and resecured to the floor), Dad hired a carpet professional to restretch the carpet, eliminating those hazardous ripples completely. In turn, this eliminated that particular fall risk for Mom.

We also had a problem when Mom and Dad visited my house where Mom would often run into the coffee table, giving herself a painful bruise on her leg. Fortunately, my parents didn't have a coffee table or other low-to-the-ground pieces of furniture in the middle of the rooms in their house.

There are many important things to consider and do when safety proofing your loved one's home to decrease the likelihood that they will fall. Periodically survey your loved one's home for common risks.

- **Trip hazards:** Remove or securely attach any items that could cause a slip, trip, or fall. This includes electric and extension cords, furniture positioned away from walls, shoes lying in the middle of the room, newspapers lying on the ground, and area or throw rugs that are not securely attached to the floor.

- **Uncarpeted floors:** Clean uncarpeted areas with no-wax cleaner only in order to minimize slippery floors.
- **Stairs:** Stairs, especially, are potentially hazardous. To prevent tripping and falling, *both indoor and outdoor* stairways should have secure handrails, and steps that are sturdy and either carpeted or equipped with safety grip strips. In addition, it's exceptionally important to have stairways well lit, especially at night.
- **Lighting:** To minimize the risk of falling, every part of the house where your loved one goes needs to have adequate lighting during the day and night.
- **Mobility aids:** Mobility aids such as canes, walkers, and bathtub transfer benches can go a long way to reduce the risk of falling. (Be sure to have a physical or occupational therapist assess whether a cane or walker is a safe addition for your loved one.)

Burns, Shocks, and Other Hazards

In addition to falling, we also worried about Mom getting burned, especially in the kitchen. As her dementia progressed, Mom started leaving dishtowels and paper products (mostly mail) on the stovetop, not noticing if the heating elements were turned on. When she started showing lapses in judgment, we knew it was time to modify kitchen appliances. Mary's husband, Mike, showed Dad how to disable the range and oven and how to easily detach (and reattach when necessary) knobs from appliances. To be on the safe side, when Mom couldn't see what he was doing, Dad started unplugging the washer and dryer and hiding the cords behind the appliances.

Actions to Take to Reduce Risk of Burns and Shock

- Disable stove and oven
- Remove knobs from appliances
- Unplug appliances and hide cords
- Cover unused outlets with outlet covers
- Set the water heater to 120 degrees Fahrenheit or less to help prevent burns from scalding water

One other key safety precaution you can take is to look for flammable objects and other items in your loved one's home that could cause a shock, burn, or other injuries, or even a fire if not properly used or supervised during use. These include such flammable objects and compounds as:

- Cigarettes, pipes, and lighters
- Gas and electric appliances
- Gas and charcoal grills
- Portable space heaters
- Heating pads and electric blankets
- Electrical cords near a water source
- Fireplaces
- Tools and machinery
- Guns, knives, and other weapons

All of the above require that your loved one be supervised when they near these devices whether they are being used or not. As an extra precaution, make sure that all smoke and carbon monoxide detectors are in good working order in the living room, kitchen, bedrooms, and other key areas.

Food Safety

Preparing and eating food both pose considerable risks for people with Alzheimer's disease. There are a number of things you can do to make food safer for your loved one.

Food Preparation

If your loved one likes to cook or prepare meals, keep sharp knives and utensils locked away. Your loved one should also be supervised in the kitchen if possible; kitchen accidents, especially cuts and burns (see above) are very common among the elderly.

Choking and Safety at Mealtime

Choking is also a major concern for people with Alzheimer's disease. The good news is that there are many precautions and interventions that can decrease the risk of your loved one choking on food:

- Always supervise meals and snacks, watching for signs of choking
- Make sure your loved one only eats when they are sitting upright and are fully awake
- Allow plenty of time for meals and snacks
- Keep mealtime calm and quiet, limiting distractions as much as possible
- Cut food into bite-sized pieces to make it easier to chew and swallow, and also to make it easier for your loved one to feed themself
- If you do notice swallowing or choking troubles, give your loved one soft foods, such as ice cream, milk shakes, soups, applesauce, or yogurt
- Make sure your loved one drinks fluids with meals and throughout the day to help with swallowing and digestion, while also minimizing the chance of dehydration

Food Spoilage

Finally, be sure to monitor foods regularly for expiration dates and spoilage.

Medication Safety

Prescription and even over-the-counter drugs pose serious risks of overdosing as well as choking.

Reducing Choking Risk with Medications

As with food, make sure your loved one is sitting upright and is fully awake when they take their medications. If they have trouble taking medication because of choking or swallowing problems, try crushing the pills to mix with food or drinks, or find out if that medication comes in liquid form.

Managing Medications Safely

Make sure that all of your loved one's drugs have been ordered or approved by their physician. Educate yourself about their medications, including dosage, frequency, benefits, and possible side effects. You or someone else you trust should supervise your loved one to make sure the correct medications are taken at the right time in the right dosage. And, of course, all medications should be safely stored and locked away.

Because your loved one might be taking many drugs at different times of the day, or even on different days, using a drug organizer and maintaining an updated chart of all medications can be extremely helpful. Also, keep track of the medications that have been discontinued and maintain a record that explains why as well as when the medication was stopped. Believe me, you'll be happy you did should that same medication ever be prescribed by another doctor.

One of the most stressful parts of caring for Mom was managing her medications, especially the last year or so she was at home. As her dementia progressed, various drugs were added or changed to manage the effects of dementia on her mood and behavior. By then, Mom's primary care physician was only treating her if she needed general care, but he was also aware of what her other doctors were prescribing for her. This simplified home management of her medications. Her dementia neurologist handled everything Alzheimer's related including dementia medications, and her primary care doctor handled her other drugs.

But we were still overwhelmed at times, checking and double-checking that all medications prescribed for her—including nonprescription medications, vitamins, and herbal supplements—were compatible. Every time there was a change to her medications, Dad had to reorganize his home pharmacy, removing discontinued medications and storing them away safely. We helped him with that and kept in close touch with Mom's pharmacist every time something was added or changed. It really did give us some peace of mind that an expert was keeping a watchful eye on her prescription and nonprescription drugs.

Other Poisoning Possibilities

While spoiled food and medications can pose threats to your loved one, there are plenty of other items in a home that can poison them as well. So, in addition to locking up medications, lock up all wine, beer, and other alcoholic beverages as well as all toxic materials such as cleaning products, flammable liquids, laundry products, paint, fertilizers, pesticides, and gasoline, among others.

If you have a pet, all pet foods and pet medications also need to be safely stored out of reach or locked away. In fact, anything that could make a person sick from consuming it needs to be securely stored.

It's also a good idea to research the plants in your house and yard. If they're considered poisonous, they should be removed.

Finally, keep emergency numbers handy. This list should include the local poison control center as well as other essential emergency numbers.

Emergency Preparedness

I wish I could tell you my family and I discussed plans for Mom in case of an emergency. But we had neither an emergency kit nor an emergency plan, and we were lucky that no serious emergency occurred while Mom was still at home. However, I look back on a situation that could have easily turned disastrous. Dad was stuck in traffic during a snowstorm. Mom was home alone. My sister Mary and I were each stuck at work. Because Dad didn't have a cell phone, we weren't able to be in contact with him to check on his progress home. Mom wasn't driving anymore, so we were relieved that she couldn't get in a car and start driving in the storm looking for Dad. But unfortunately, as she watched the outside landscape transform in the snow, there was no one at home to watch her and reassure her that she was safe and that Dad would be home soon. Luckily, Mom did know how to answer the phone. I can't tell you how many times I called her to check in until Dad got home safely. She sounded anxious, but thankfully, didn't give the slightest hint that she would do anything risky to her safety.

In hindsight, it would have been wise to acknowledge the possibility of an event like that and plan for it in advance. Our plan might have included things like each of us keeping a phone list of Mom and Dad's neighbors should we need to reach them, notifying their neighbors of Mom's condition, and getting Dad a cell phone. In fact this incident was a wake-up call and incentive enough to finally get Dad a cell phone!

There are a number of important things you can do to prepare for an emergency:
- Make sure everyone has a cell phone
- Post a list of emergency and other important numbers and your loved one's home address near each of their phones
- Keep a copy of that list with you at all times

- Prepare an emergency kit and emergency plan (details on what to include can be found at www.alz.org/care/ alzheimers-dementia-disaster-preparedness.asp).
- Hide a spare house key near the outside of your loved one's house in case you get locked out or someone else needs to gain immediate access
- Have your loved one wear an ID bracelet in case they get separated from you on an outing or they wander from home on their own

Also, seriously consider getting your loved one a home monitoring device or alarms to alert you (or others) to falls, injuries, or other emergencies, especially if they live alone. But this is also important if they live with a spouse or other caregiver. Falls and other injuries can happen out of sight and hearing or in the middle of the night. There are also monitoring devices that work in cars and outside the home. This is especially important if your loved one still drives or if they wander away from home.

Wandering from Home

The effects of dementia can make people behave in ways that are different and unexpected from when they were healthy (see Chapter 7: Coping with Disturbing Behaviors and Emotions). And wandering from home on their own is one of them. We've all seen gut-wrenching news stories about missing people with dementia.

A counselor at the Alzheimer's Association gave me some wonderful advice that won't prevent your loved one from wandering away from home but that could assist you should they wander: Inform your loved one's neighbors as well as the local police and fire departments of their diagnosis. Knowing that a cognitively impaired person is living at a particular address can help identify them if they are found wandering or are reported missing. Having this information is also important in case of a fire or other neighborhood emergency.

There are several other measures you can put in place to minimize the chance that your loved one will wander away from home:

- Make sure all outside doors and windows are locked
- Install hardware that limits how far a window can be opened
- Install alarms and bells to alert you if your loved one leaves the house through a window or door they shouldn't be using
- Label all articles of clothing with your loved one's name in case they do wander away from the home
- Lock all motor vehicles when not in use, and lock away the keys
- Get your loved one an ID bracelet or electronic-tracking device, especially if they have wandered in the past
- Supervise your loved one appropriately, even if this means never leaving them home alone

Making Decisions about Leaving Your Loved One Home Alone

I think one of the hardest decisions to make regarding dementia can be determining when it's no longer safe for your loved one to be left alone. If your loved one wanders, the decision is cut and dried: they should definitely not be left alone. But what if wandering isn't a problem, and you've proofed your home to the best of your abilities? The best way to determine when that time has come is to be observant. Your loved one will show signs that will alert you to real or potential safety risks if they are left on their own.

For example, your loved one might forget how to:
- Turn off the water in the kitchen or bathroom
- Turn off the stove
- Turn lights on and off
- Make or answer phone calls

If you're still uncertain, ask yourself the following questions:
- Do you ever worry about their safety when your loved one is alone?
- Do you frequently have to check on your loved one when you're not with them?
- Does your loved one attempt to get into locked cabinets or rooms?
- Is frequent assistance or supervision needed during the day or night?

A *yes* to any of these questions is a good reason to no longer leave your loved one home alone.

Also consider the following question: is your loved one able to identify an emergency situation (a fire, flood, burglary, etc.) and take the appropriate steps to secure their own safety by calling 911 or promptly exiting the home? If the answer is *no,* for both their safety and your peace of mind, they should not be allowed to be home alone.

Another important consideration is that the dementia-related behaviors your loved one exhibits with others will most likely be present when they are left alone. These include aggression and anger, anxiety and agitation, depression, hallucinations, memory loss, confusion, suspicion, and delusions (see Chapter 7: Coping with Disturbing Behaviors and Emotions). If any of these or other behaviors pose a safety risk (such as punching a mirror or wall), your loved one should not be left alone.

If you decide that your loved one can safely be left home alone, be sure to regularly evaluate the safety points above. But realistically speaking, at some point, your loved one will need constant supervision.

Driving Dangers

As you can see from the above, deciding to leave your loved one home alone is a decision that can have major safety consequences. But an even more critical decision is whether or not to allow them to drive. This not only impacts their safety, but that of fellow passengers, other drivers, and pedestrians as well.

Mom's driving was one of the most serious safety issues we faced. We first became aware that driving was becoming a problem one day when she was going to stop at a store to pick up some ginger ale because my son and I were sick. An hour and a half after we discussed this plan on the phone, I hadn't heard from Mom and became very concerned. It normally would have taken her thirty minutes to get from her house to mine, including the brief stop at the store. When Mom finally arrived, she admitted that she had gotten lost, but she couldn't provide me with any details of what exactly had happened. I found it both disconcerting and interesting that she told me about getting lost so matter-of-factly—there was neither anxiety nor concern in her voice or attitude.

Although we were becoming concerned about her driving, we didn't try to get Mom to stop at that point. As far as we knew, Mom had never had an accident or any other driving-related safety issue, so we believed it was OK to let her drive short distances from home.

The final straw, for me at least, came a few months later. At that point I no longer felt comfortable having her babysit my then five-year-old son without my father being present. The plan was for me to drop Matthew off at my parents' house so that I could go to work. When we arrived at the house, Mom was home alone. Although Dad was expected home any minute, I had an uncomfortable feeling about leaving Matthew alone with Mom that I could not shake. But truthfully, I also felt pressure to get to work on time. So I said to Mom, "Please don't take Matthew anywhere until Dad gets home." She became upset and responded by saying that she was perfectly capable of driving Matthew somewhere.

Cursing the predicament I found myself in, I turned to my kindergarten-aged child and put the responsibility on his small shoulders. I told Matthew not to get in the car with his grandma unless his grandpa was with them. He said he wouldn't. But when I left, Mom suggested they take a trip to get ice cream. Dad came home a few minutes later to find the house empty. Within minutes, Mom came pulling up with Matthew saying that she had forgotten her purse. As soon as I got to work, I called Dad to check on Matthew, and he nonchalantly relayed the ice-cream story to me. As they had arrived home safely, all was well from Dad's perspective. But I was very upset when I heard what had happened. Mom's driving haunted me. It would have been bad enough if something happened to her while she was driving. But it was unbearable to think of Mom causing injury or worse to someone else, especially Matthew.

Our family had countless conversations and disagreements about Mom's driving during that year. Dad and I had the strongest—and most opposing—opinions. While Dad did the driving for both of them whenever possible, his position was that Mom should still be allowed to drive because she only drove to familiar places and had not been involved in any kind of accident. However, his arguments didn't shake my belief that we had a responsibility to get Mom off the road in the name of safety.

Did this difference of opinion mean that my father disregarded the possible danger Mom's continued driving posed just to keep the peace and status quo in their home? Absolutely not. Dad really believed Mom's driving was already limited and that she was a safe driver during the small amount of time she was behind the wheel. One issue I failed to acknowledge was that if she didn't drive anymore, it would be a loss for Dad. In all the years my parents had been married, Mom had been a self-sufficient and contributing member of their partnership. The effects of dementia were radically changing that dynamic. Mom was becoming more dependent on Dad, yet another concrete example of his increasing responsibility for her.

Looking to solidify my position, I scheduled a meeting for me and Dad with a counselor at the Alzheimer's Association to discuss Mom's driving. Dad attended reluctantly. "You have a moral responsibility to get the car keys from your wife," the counselor said. She further explained that part of the issue of driving with dementia is not that people with dementia can't read the word *stop* on a stop sign, it's that the word *stop* might no longer have that meaning to them all the time, if at all.

According to the Alzheimer's Association, "[d]riving is a complex activity that requires quick thinking and reactions, as well as good perceptual abilities."[1] From this statement it follows that driving is something that should be avoided by people diagnosed with Alzheimer's disease at a certain point. In other words, it's better to be safe than sorry. That said, each individual case is different.

Help for Making Decisions about Driving

If you're uncertain about your loved one's ability to drive safely, there are important warning signs of unsafe driving that can help you decide. Your loved one should not be driving if they:

- Drive either too fast or too slow
- Forget how to find familiar places
- Get confused or angry while driving
- Ignore traffic signs or respond inappropriately to them

- Respond slowly or make bad decisions when in driving traffic

In addition, stay alert for new scratches and dents on your loved one's car. Talk to your loved one when you start noticing signs of unsafe driving, and express your concerns by providing concrete examples if possible. Expect this to be a difficult conversation as they might be unaware of their unsafe driving practices and might feel threatened by your *accusations*. If at all possible, include your loved one in the decision to stop driving.

It might also be useful to arrange to have a driving evaluation through the American Occupational Therapy Association (AOTA). Because such an evaluation is conducted by an objective third party, it might be better received by your loved one than your opinion alone. In particular, reaction time and decision making are evaluated. Based on the results of the evaluation, recommendations are made. The evaluator (an occupational therapist) can offer strategies to improve your loved one's driving safety or can recommend that your loved one stop driving altogether. If your loved one does not have a driving evaluation through the AOTA, your state's department of motor vehicles might require your loved one to retake a driving test. It helps to become educated on your state's driving regulations. The Alzheimer's Association can provide you with this information. Another option is to have your loved one's physician tell them that it's unsafe for them to drive and write a *do not drive prescription.*

If you're still undecided about whether your loved one should be allowed to drive, or are meeting resistance, there are some tactics you can try to discourage them from driving. For example, always offer to be the driver. You can tell them that you found a new, better route to take or that it would be a good chance for them to enjoy being a passenger for a change. If you decide that it's dangerous for your loved one to drive but can't dissuade them, lock away the keys, or take more drastic measures such as having a mechanic disable the car or even putting the car up for sale. It also helps to enlist support from your loved one's family and friends. They can help discourage your loved one from driving as well as pitching in when driving help is needed.

Sooner or later, you'll have to shift all driving responsibilities to family, friends, or others. You can use a transportation service for senior citizens, call a taxi, or use a car service such as Uber. Also, use home-delivery services whenever possible for prescriptions, food, or other necessities.

When dealing with driving issues, always be mindful of the feelings your loved one might be experiencing including confusion, anger, fear, and loss. This issue is tough to confront as a caregiver, but it might be equally if not more difficult for your loved one with dementia.

After meeting with the counselor, we agreed that it was time for Mom to stop driving. We tried various ways to persuade her to stop, but in the end, we simply took her car key off her key chain. She never once asked where it was. Well, to be honest, it wasn't really *that* simple. Mom continued to believe that she could drive. We had always shared driving duties whenever we went out together. Amazingly, she continued to always offer to drive whenever she and I went out. Because we had always alternated who would do the driving, I got around it by telling her that because as she had driven the last time, it was now my turn to drive. This approach worked. And because Dad was semi-retired and home most of the time, he was available to drive Mom whenever and wherever she wanted to go.

Conclusion

I bet you'll notice in the next chapter the connection between the behaviors that are commonly exhibited by those with Alzheimer's disease and how those behaviors can impact your loved one's safety. As with so many aspects of Alzheimer's caregiving, learning how to best manage the challenging behaviors your loved one exhibits requires an ability to alter your approach as the disease progresses.

Resources

General Safety Information

▶ **ADEAR (The Alzheimer's Disease Education and Referral Center)**
Several publications on home safety and driver safety are available to order or download and print.
www.nia.nih.gov/alzheimers/topics/caregiving

▶ **The Alzheimer's Association 1–800–272–3900**
The Alzheimer's Association offers numerous pamphlets and other publications on safety issues that can be found at your local Alzheimer's Association or online to be viewed or downloaded and printed.
www.alz.org/alzheimers_disease_publications_safety.asp

▶ **Family Caregiver Alliance**
"Assistive Technology" introduces the topics of independent-living aids and adaptive equipment as it relates to your loved one's safety.
www.caregiver.org/fact-sheets

▶ **MedicAlert + Alzheimer's Association Safe Return**
This 24-hour, nationwide alert system provides an additional safety net for people with dementia who wander or have a medical emergency. Information on the ID bracelet or pendant includes their personalized information and the 24-hour emergency, toll-free number for MedicAlert + Safe Return.
www.alz.org/care/dementia-medic-alert-safe-return.asp

Driving and Driver Safety

▶ **ADEAR (The Alzheimer's Disease Education and Referral Center)**
Several publications on home safety and driver safety are available to order or download and print.
www.nia.nih.gov/alzheimers/topics/caregiving

▶ **The American Occupational Therapy Association**
Research local driving specialists who can perform a driver evaluation on your loved one with Alzheimer's disease.
www.aota.org/Practice/Productive-Aging/Driving.aspx

▶ **The Eldercare Locator**
The Eldercare Locator has publications on older driver safety and offers links to national information and resources on transportation.
www.eldercare.gov/eldercare.net/public/resources/topic/Transportation.aspx

▶ **Family Caregiver Alliance**
"Dementia and Driving" is a publication to help prepare you for the many considerations when deciding that it's time for your loved one to stop driving.
www.caregiver.org/fact-sheets

▶ **Peter Rabins Alzheimer's Family Support Center**
"Driving—Memory and Alzheimer's Disease"
www.youtube.com/watch?v=cE84bWGWcQo&feature=youtu.be

Transportation Services

▶ **The Community Resource Finder**
The Community Resource Finder through the
Alzheimer's Association allows you to access
comprehensive listings of transportation services for
your loved one.
www.communityresourcefinder.org/

▶ **The Eldercare Locator**
From this page you can search for transportation
resources in your area.
www.eldercare.gov/eldercare.net/public/resources/
topic/Transportation.aspx

▶ **The National Highway Traffic Safety Administration**
NHTSA's section on older drivers offers numerous
downloadable publications.
www.nhtsa.gov/road-safety/older-drivers

Seven

Coping with Disturbing Behaviors and Emotions

About a week before Christmas each year, Mom's nursing home hosts an afternoon holiday party for the residents and their families. There are music, refreshments, gifts, and a visit from Santa. It's very festive and a nice way for us and other families to celebrate the holidays with our loved ones. The festivities, for the most part, take place in the atrium, which is outside Mom's memory-care unit. However, Santa and his helpers do stroll through her unit to deliver gifts. Family members can choose to take their loved ones to the atrium for the party or not. During Mom's first Christmas in the nursing home we decided to participate in the party by bringing Mom to the atrium. If memory serves, one of my sisters or my dad attended the party with Mom. It was noisy, busy, crowded, and festive—something Mom would have loved pre-dementia.

When I arrived for dinner later that day, I found Mom pacing the halls in a very anxious and agitated mood. Looking for a reason to explain Mom's foul mood, I asked the nurse. She told me that she had most likely become overstimulated by the party earlier in the day. I spent the next hour trying to calm Mom, using many of the techniques I describe later in this chapter but without success. Because Mom wouldn't sit down for dinner, I followed her around, handing her food from her dinner plate, or spoon feeding her in an attempt to get her to eat something.

Finally, the nurse stopped me and said, "Amy, this is not what your Mom needs right now. We will not let her go hungry. When she calms down, we'll give her something to eat. But when your Mom gets like this, she needs to be able to work it out. And she will, but she needs the space to do it."

I wanted to share this story with you, not to expose my limitations as an Alzheimer's caregiver, but rather to clearly illustrate that sometimes there really isn't a great solution to your loved one's dementia-related behaviors. Nonetheless, upon further reflection, I realized there was something we could have done that might have prevented Mom from becoming so upset in the first place. We could have taken into account her limitations due to Alzheimer's disease and respected them. Since that first holiday party, we still celebrate Christmas with Mom but in a different way. Before we visit, we pick up some punch and food from the party and eat it with Mom in the comfort of her memory-care unit.

Because Alzheimer's disease gradually destroys a person's memory, ability to think clearly, and even perform routine daily tasks, it's no wonder that my mother and others suffering from Alzheimer's disease get confused, depressed, angry, and agitated, in addition to displaying other disturbing behaviors. Think of how difficult it must be for them to try to function and relate to others and the world around them when their memory and ability to think, understand, and communicate are being ravaged by the effects of this devastating disease. These internal, troubling changes—as well as the resulting inevitable changes in their relationships, daily lives, and environment—can cause a whole host of atypical behaviors and emotions including repetition, rummaging, depression, and even physical aggression, to name a few. These and other troublesome behaviors might seem to come out of the blue, but specific causes can often be identified. And when they are, finding solutions to these behaviors becomes much easier.

My family and I tried to prepare ahead of time for certain behavioral issues we would likely encounter with Mom's advancing dementia. However, there were others we couldn't anticipate, and as a result, we had to react to some of the disturbing behaviors Mom exhibited as they developed. While that wasn't ideal and I wouldn't recommend that style of management, it's given me much to ponder in hindsight. Specifically, what we could have done differently to possibly influence a better outcome for Mom. Below, I describe our experiences trying to cope with Mom's behavior issues and some of the tactics I would attempt now, having the luxury of hindsight.

Repetitive Behaviors

Without a doubt, the most prevalent and longest lasting of Mom's behavior problems was repetition. It felt like Mom verbally repeated herself almost constantly for years because, in fact, she did!

While repetitive behaviors can occur at any stage of Alzheimer's disease, it was the first unusual behavior that surfaced in Mom. She repeated questions, stories, or actions over and over again. "Are you dating anyone?" became the question I was repeatedly asked for a few years every time Mom and I were together. While she hasn't asked that question in several years, a repetitive behavior that continues with Mom to this day is pacing. She used to pace throughout her home, especially late in the day and sometimes through the night as other sundowning behaviors surfaced. To me, it seemed Mom was just too agitated to be able to sit peacefully and relax. She is now in a wheelchair most of the time, but that has not curtailed her pacing in the least. Truthfully, she seems most content when she cruises through the halls of her unit, and fortunately she is given the freedom to do so by the nursing home staff. I think the difference between Mom's pacing in the evening and at night at home and her pacing now is that when she was still living at home, Dad didn't feel safe falling asleep with her up and unsupervised. In the nursing home, the staff are awake twenty-four hours a day and are able to keep an eye on her as she roams.

This peculiar behavior—and others as well—is caused by Alzheimer's-related changes in the brain and can best be managed by trying to find a specific reason or precipitating factor for the repetitive behavior. If it surfaces around certain people or surroundings, or at a particular time of the day, you can try to avoid those stimuli and find something distracting and calming to do instead.

You can also try turning a repetitive behavior into a positive activity. For example, if your loved one repeatedly rubs his or her hand up and down a window, give them a cloth to wash the window with. But, most importantly, no matter how many times they repeat a question, comment, or behavior, try to respond calmly and without any sign of annoyance.

We never did discover a tactic to decrease the frequency of Mom's repetitive questions and statements. However, through trial and error, we did learn how to handle the situation without upsetting her. This involved careful communication, from the words we chose to our facial expressions and body language. If we responded to Mom's repetitive questions and statements with patience, her mood generally stayed calm and pleasant. But if we called her out for repeating things or asking the same questions, or if we responded with exasperation either in word or attitude, she would become very agitated. We then had to deal with an additional disturbing behavior—anger.

Mom's anger manifested itself verbally, and luckily, not physically. She usually responded to what she perceived as criticism by going on the defensive and verbally lashing out. It was bad enough that we noticed a deficiency (her repetitive behavior), but the fact that we pointed it out to her was what got her so angry.

If repetition was the behavior we dealt with the longest, aggression, anger, agitation, sleep issues, and sundowning, all of which are discussed below, were the issues that challenged us the most.

Anger, Aggression, Anxiety, and Agitation

Anger and aggressive behaviors, which are common in people with Alzheimer's disease, might be expressed verbally by yelling or physically by hitting, pushing, and even biting. While being put on the defensive can cause anger and aggression, frustration is probably the most common cause. Forgetting a close relative's name or important facts or being unable to perform simple tasks, especially when pushed by others, can make your loved one feel very frustrated. Their frustration can quickly turn to anger, which they might take out on others or even themselves.

However, not all frustration leads to anger and aggression. Frustration might make your loved one nervous and anxious where they suffer internally rather than acting out externally. Because it's not always easy to determine how someone with Alzheimer's disease will react to frustration, the best thing to do is try to control or avoid frustration in the first place by not making unnecessary demands.

Any change in your loved one's physical environment, living arrangement, caregiver, or routine is bound to be upsetting and can also lead to anxiety, anger, aggression, and other disturbing behaviors. The same goes for traveling or hospitalizations.

Your physical presence and reassurance during these changes and transitions is especially important.

Anxiety and aggression can also be set off by too much noise or too many people in the room. On the other hand, feeling lonely and not having enough people around can be just as bad. Finding the right balance is key ... and challenging. In general, however, try to keep a calm, quiet, uncluttered environment and limit the number of people in the room. Relaxing music and activities, such as a quiet walk or a massage, might help.

It's also important to pay attention to your loved one's physical condition. They might become agitated and aggressive, or display other troublesome behaviors, if they've soiled themselves, are constipated, are in pain, or don't get enough sleep. These behaviors can also be related to medication side effects, so be sure to discuss them with your loved one's physician.

Sleep Problems and Sundowning

Beginning in the late afternoon and into the night, many people with Alzheimer's disease experience sundowning symptoms, which can include agitation, pacing, irritability, and disorientation. Alzheimer's disease can cause a disruption in the body's internal clock, making it difficult to distinguish day from night. One solution is to make sure your loved one is exposed to natural light every day. Also adequate indoor lighting is important not just for safety reasons (see Chapter 6: Safety First) but because dark rooms and shadows can cause your loved one to become confused, disoriented, and frightened. You can minimize shadows by keeping their home well lit during the evening and at night, as well as keeping curtains and blinds closed at dusk. Also, limit both caffeine and stimulating activities in the late afternoon and early evening. Because certain medications can cause sleep disturbances, it's important to discuss any sleep problems with your loved one's physician.

Mom exhibited sundowning behaviors for at least a couple of years before her move to the nursing home. Looking back, Dad managed it on his own. Unless there was an incident he shared with us, my sisters and I were not aware of the extent of Mom's sleep disruption. However, we came face to face with Mom's sundowning behaviors while Dad was briefly away from home. Mom and I were watching TV one evening and she was very antsy, unable to sit still for more than a moment or two. Pacing from room to room, Mom would return, saying, "Come on. Let's go!" But she was unable to tell me where she wanted to go or why. As I was formulating a plan in my mind to calm her anxiety, she returned to the family room. Although it was late summer, she was dressed in her winter coat, hat, scarf, and gloves. Anxiously, she pleaded with me, "Come on. Let's go!" So I led her to the front door and opened it. It was dark outside, and I prayed Mom could comprehend that darkness indicated nighttime. I said, "Mom, it's too late to go anywhere tonight. Let's go tomorrow morning." Even though she seemed satisfied with my explanation, her anxiety didn't magically vanish. It took some time. I helped her take off the winter attire, turned off the TV, and prepared a snack for her in the kitchen. Slowly, very slowly, her anxiety and agitation decreased.

At the time, I didn't have a plan B if plan A failed. But hindsight is twenty-twenty. Knowing that Mom usually responded positively to movement or motion, I could have said: "OK, let's go." Then I could have taken her for a drive to see if changing the environment would have been calming to her. Nonetheless, looking back, the only consistent remedy for Mom's behavior problems was sleep. If she slept well, these odd behaviors would retreat somewhat until later the next day. If not, we did our best to deal with them until she slept again.

Confusion

People with Alzheimer's disease often become very confused, which is understandable given their memory problems. They might not recognize familiar people, places, or even everyday items, which results in confusion. Memory problems and confusion, as well as most behavioral changes seen in people with Alzheimer's disease, are caused by progressive damage to brain cells. But changes in living arrangements, routines, or caregivers, as well as infections and other illnesses, can also cause or exacerbate confusion.

As Mom's dementia progressed, her confusion became more pronounced. Predictability was a big part of managing Mom's confusion. Dad established a predictable routine for their daily lives that, I think, helped Mom feel safe and less confused. For example, they went to the same restaurant every day for breakfast. It was helpful that the staff got to know both of my parents well and that they were aware of Mom's dementia. Over time they became very comfortable with how best to communicate with her.

Mom often would get confused when we were offering directions to assist her in completing a task. Not surprisingly, though, communication was key (see Chapter 4: Communication Strategies). In giving directions, we needed to use simple and concise wording, as well as words, names, and phrases that were familiar to her while also answering her questions with very simple answers and explanations. If we failed to do any of these things, Mom would get very confused. When she did become confused, showing her compassion, care, and concern with our words, tone of voice, and body language helped considerably.

It's also important to live in the moment with your loved one; whatever time or place they are focused on, engage them about those memories. For example, if they mention that their long-deceased spouse will be getting home from work any minute, rather than reminding your loved one that their spouse died long ago, respond by saying something like, "I hope so-and-so had a good day at work." Trying to bring them back to the present or your reality will only confuse (and possibly upset) them.

Rummaging and Hoarding

Rummaging and **hoarding** are among the more unusual behaviors seen in people with Alzheimer's disease. These odd behaviors are also the result of Alzheimer's-related changes in the brain. Rummaging involves searching though drawers, closets, cabinets, mailboxes, and even refrigerators for something the person might think is missing. Hoarding, which might or might not be associated with rummaging, involves collecting or hiding objects or both.

Both rummaging and hoarding can be problematic if your loved one finds or hides important or valuable items or documents and then forgets where they put them. These behaviors are potentially dangerous if what they find or collect are dangerous objects such as knives, poisonous substances such as cleaning fluids, or spoiled food (see Chapter 6: Safety First). Besides locking away valuables, dangerous objects, and poisonous substances in drawers, safes, or special containers, there are several other strategies that can help you manage these behaviors:

- Lock rooms that your loved one might find especially tempting such as the kitchen, attic, or garage
- Lock or move the mailbox to a secure spot if you suspect mail is being hidden or thrown out
- Learn where your loved one prefers to hide things and check those places regularly

- Because trash cans can be especially tempting for both rummaging and hoarding, keep them out of sight and check the contents before disposing of them

And finally, set aside a special space—whether it's a corner of a room or an entire room—where your loved one can freely and safely rummage or hoard. Then provide a basket or a desk or dresser with drawers filled with clothing or other safe items for rummaging or hoarding.

Hallucinations and Delusions

Hallucinations

One of the most disturbing behaviors to witness in your loved one is **hallucinations**. Hallucinations can affect all of their five senses: they might see, hear, feel, taste, or smell things that aren't there. In addition to being caused by Alzheimer's-related changes in the brain, hallucinations can be triggered by some physical problems, especially kidney and bladder infections, dehydration, and pain. Ear and eye problems as well as alcohol and drugs (both illicit and prescription) can also cause hallucinations. If you notice your loved one hallucinating, have their doctor rule out medical causes.

Also, try the following approaches:

- Get their attention and reassure them with gentle pats or words
- Distract them by taking a walk or moving to another room
- Turn their attention to enjoyable activities
- Minimize shadows by keeping all rooms and areas well lit
- Turn off or lower sounds that can be misinterpreted, such as the TV or air conditioner
- Cover or remove mirrors if your loved one sees strangers in them

Hallucinations can be benign or even pleasurable. But they can also be very frightening. One night, Mom awoke in the middle of the night and I found her at the top of the stairs, visibly frightened. As I approached her, it was obvious that she believed someone had gotten into the house with malicious intent. I thought about taking Mom downstairs to show her that all was well. But short of me physically forcing her down the stairs, she was not about to take one step in that direction. Instead, I quietly coaxed her back to bed and spent the next hour with my arms around her, comforting and reassuring her the best I could until she was relaxed enough to fall back asleep.

Mom continues to have visual hallucinations in the nursing home. Focusing on something or someone in front of her, she reaches for things that are not there and tosses items gently, as if to someone she sees who does not exist for the rest of us. Thankfully, these hallucinations do not seem to cause her anxiety or agitation. Because of that, I don't intervene or worry.

Delusions

Whether or not your loved one actually hallucinates, they might become suspicious and delusional about people or events. **Delusions** are false ideas that, in spite of proof to the contrary, are strongly believed. The cause of delusions and paranoid ideas is similar to that of hallucinations. In addition, because of their decline in memory, people with Alzheimer's disease might have difficulty trusting others. They might believe that people, including friends or relatives, are stealing from them or even trying to poison them. Gentle reassurance and the same strategies used for hallucinations can be helpful. Also, don't let your loved one watch or listen to programs, shows, or movies that are violent or otherwise upsetting as they could misinterpret those as reality or even a direct threat.

My mom experienced an ongoing delusion that was most prevalent late in the day. Mom has always been a devout Catholic, which is relevant to the story only because she had strong ideas and convictions about certain things that could be traced back to her religious beliefs. One evening at their home, Mom told Dad that it was time for him to go home. When Dad responded by saying he was already at home, Mom became upset. As hard as he tried, he could not convince her that they were married and it was okay for them to be living together. This back and forth went on for a while with Dad becoming increasingly frustrated and Mom increasingly agitated. Sometime in the middle of this heated exchange, Mom jumped up and told Dad she needed to call 911 to report that he was trying to force her to live with him before they were lawfully married. Exasperated, Dad said, "Fine. Do it!" not thinking that Mom was capable of carrying out her threat. She was! After she called 911, Mom left the house, shouting out for help. A neighbor heard her cry for help and approached her. The police arrived as Dad was explaining everything to the neighbor. Because the police officers had no prior knowledge of Mom's dementia, they lectured her and Dad on the inappropriate use of 911. Mom's response to anything the police officers had to say was, "I didn't do it!" As discussed in the prior chapter on safety, it would have been helpful for the police and Dad's neighbors to be aware of Mom's Alzheimer's diagnosis.

While that was not the last time Mom became fixated on that particular delusion, it never escalated to that level again. Since then, I've thought about how that situation could have been handled better. I've wondered if Dad could have responded to Mom's delusion by agreeing to leave, kissing her goodnight, telling her he would see her later, leaving the house for fifteen minutes, and then returning home as if from a day at work. I'll never know if the outcome would have been any different, but in hindsight, it would have been worth trying.

Illness, Pain, and Behavior

I can't emphasize enough the importance of informing your loved one's physician about any behavioral changes you notice. And the sooner the better. The myriad of medical problems that typically plague the elderly, such as pain and infections, can even have more profound physical, emotional, and behavioral effects on people suffering from Alzheimer's disease.

For example, Mom was very social, physically spry, and conversational even after she was diagnosed with Alzheimer's disease. But quite suddenly, her gait became unsteady to such a degree that she had to hold onto something or have someone support her while she walked. Her language skills also declined markedly—she wasn't making much sense and she was very confused. The change in her alarmed us greatly until Dad shared with us that she had been battling a gastrointestinal virus. Then I remembered reading that when people with dementia are sick or in pain, their behavior is often affected as well. Within a couple of days after she was treated, Mom had rebounded completely to her pre-illness self.

I also can't stress enough the importance of paying attention to your loved one's subtle as well as not-so-subtle sudden behavior changes. The staff at Mom's nursing home routinely search for a cause of even minor increases in her irritability or agitation level that last more than a day (without any overt signs of illness or pain being present). The few times they were alerted by what I considered a minute change in Mom's behavior, they always found a physical cause. Once treated, Mom would soon return to her old self, relatively speaking. That said, as Mom continues to decline from the effects of Alzheimer's disease, it not only takes her longer to bounce back from an injury or illness, she doesn't usually rebound entirely.

General Strategies

Any success we found managing Mom's dementia-related behaviors was preceded by much trial and error. As mentioned above, one of the interventions we successfully used to manage dementia-related behaviors is one that you, undoubtedly, already use: effective communication (see Chapter 4: Communication Strategies). As Alzheimer's caregivers, we've been experimenting with communication techniques since our loved ones were first diagnosed. And, most likely, you already know which ones tend to elicit a positive interaction with your loved one, and which ones to avoid. In my experience, effective communication is the singularly most impactful strategy we can employ to manage the troublesome behaviors associated with Alzheimer's disease.

The home environment matters too. Another way to manage many of the behaviors associated with Alzheimer's disease is to maintain an environment that is safe, tidy, and free of chaos. Establishing daily and evening routines that are consistent and structured can be immensely helpful.

Also, try to:

- Keep familiar objects and photographs around the house
- Be mindful that crowds of people can be overwhelming
- Keep noise and clutter to a minimum
- Keep evenings peaceful and quiet

In addition, try to identify what are troublesome and overwhelming situations for your loved one and then limit their exposure to those situations. When a disturbing behavior does surface, look for a specific trigger. What happened right before can help clue you in to the cause.

Because illness, pain, discomfort (such as constipation or a soiled undergarment), or some other stressor (such as fatigue) are all possible causes of troublesome behaviors, rule them out.

Manage fatigue by making sure your loved one gets enough sleep at night and by building quiet times and naps into the day, especially in between activities. And be sure to report any sign of illness to your loved one's physician.

Coping with Holidays

Holidays are bittersweet for many Alzheimer's caregivers. The happy memories of the past contrast with the difficulties of the present, and extra demands on time and energy can seem overwhelming. Finding a balance between rest and activity can help. Try the following strategies from the National Institute on Aging for keeping holidays manageable for yourself and your loved one:[1]

- Keep or adapt family traditions that are important to you. Include the person with Alzheimer's disease as much as possible.
- Recognize that things will be different, and be realistic about what you can do.
- Encourage friends and family to visit. Limit the number of visitors at one time, and try to schedule visits during the time of day when the person is at his or her best.
- Avoid crowds, changes in routine, and strange places that might cause confusion or agitation.
- Do your best to enjoy yourself. Try to find time for the holiday things you like to do.
- Ask a friend or family member to spend time with the person while you are out.
- At larger gatherings such as weddings or family reunions, try to have a space available where the person can rest, be alone, or spend some time with a small number of people, if needed.

Conclusion

The behaviors associated with Alzheimer's disease can be extremely challenging to say the least. In my family's experience, we found many tactics that made Mom's disturbing behaviors manageable for quite a long time. Ultimately, though, it was these behaviors that proved to be the final straw for us. Mom got to a point (or past it) where she needed care different from what we could provide (see Chapter 9: Getting the Best Care for Your Loved One).

The last few weeks before Mom had to be admitted to a hospital and subsequently moved to a nursing home, her behavior became even more erratic and difficult to control. My sister Mary and I alternated shifts to help Dad with evening time, which was when Mom was at her worst. Fortunately, our sister Barb was moving back to Cincinnati from Los Angeles during this time. She was scheduled to arrive on a Sunday morning about a week before Christmas. Mary and I joked that we would give Barb a day to recover from the jet lag and then assign her to Monday evening duty. It's not as funny in the retelling, but it sure provided Mary and me with some much-needed laughter at a stressful time.

Besides the extra help Barb could provide, she contributed a fresh perspective as well. She had last seen Mom at Thanksgiving, and things had really gone downhill since then. Her reaction? "This is insane! We can't keep doing this!" My response? "Yeah, I know." Mary and I had just kept saying, "I guess we'll know when we can't handle it anymore."

In hindsight, of course, we had reached a point where the situation had gotten too big for us to handle. We knew things were not going well, but we were not aware enough to realize that we were not really managing Mom's behaviors in the best way possible, if at all. After all, we had been able to handle Mom's behaviors fairly well over the previous several years. The difference now, though, was that nothing we tried was successful or effective. And while we were working closely with Mom's doctor, he never saw her at her worst (she *always* slept the night before an appointment with him!), and we didn't convey to him that Mom was unmanageable or that we couldn't care for her anymore. We thought we were managing the best we could, given the circumstances.

Unfortunately, as Alzheimer's disease progresses, the behaviors associated with dementia usually become more prevalent and consequently, more stressful for both you and your loved one. So it's important to notify your loved one's physician as these behaviors surface and to routinely evaluate how they are being managed. Whether your loved one is at home or in a nursing home, mentioning any behavioral changes to their physician or medical staff is not only good for your loved ones, but for you as well. Dealing with their behavioral problems on your own only adds to the stress you experience as a caregiver.

After discussing Alzheimer's communication struggles, safety issues, and dementia-related behaviors in the last three chapters, it seems like a good time to introduce the next chapter, "Caregiver Survival." Hopefully, you will come away with some ideas to lighten your caregiving load and an acknowledgment that you deserve some time for yourself on a regular basis.

Resources

Help Dealing with Disturbing Behaviors

▶ **The Alzheimer's Association** 1–800–272–3900
This page discusses depression and Alzheimer's symptoms, diagnosis, and treatment. It also describes Alzheimer's behaviors with possible causes, as well as tips to prevent each behavior and ways to respond when a behavior surfaces.
www.alz.org/care/alzheimers-dementia-stages-behaviors.asp

▶ **ADEAR (The Alzheimer's Disease Education and Referral Center)**
There are several publications available to order or to download and print that address the behaviors associated with Alzheimer's disease.
www.nia.nih.gov/alzheimers/topics/caregiving

▶ **Family Caregiver Alliance**
"Caregiver's Guide to Understanding Dementia Behaviors" offers many suggestions on how to manage the behaviors common to people with dementia.
www.caregiver.org/health-issues/dementia

▶ **Peter Rabins Alzheimer's Family Support Center**
"Behaviors—Memory and Alzheimer's Disease" (video)
www.youtube.com/watch?v=JuıqGlJVaAA&feature=youtu.be

Eight

Caregiver Survival

As you can see from the last chapter, disturbing behaviors are bound to take a heavy toll on caregivers. They certainly did on my family and me, and I wish we had been better prepared. It wasn't until I started examining and researching the issues that Alzheimer's caregivers face that I was able to identify the two that, in my opinion, are absolutely crucial to making the caregiving experience less overwhelming. One is effective communication, which was covered in detail in Chapter 4 (Communication Strategies): successfully communicating with your loved one will make caregiving less stressful. The other is safety, the subject of Chapter 6 (Safety First): examining your loved one's home environment and making ongoing adjustments as the disease progresses will relieve some caregiving stress by reducing the chances of falls, burns, and other injuries.

Even if you are already addressing these two crucial issues, the fact is, you will still experience stress as a caregiver. It's also far too easy for caregivers to become isolated from the people and activities that have always been important them. This only adds to the stress of being a caregiver. As easy as it is to put all your focus on your loved one, addressing your own stress is key to being a successful caregiver. The focus of this chapter is on taking care of yourself and getting the help you need and deserve, as well as staying connected to others.

Caregiver Stress

While caregiving can be exceptionally rewarding, the stress of being a caregiver cannot be overstated. And that stress is especially high for women as well as for Alzheimer's and dementia caregivers (most of whom are women). Common signs of stress include the following:

- Anger
- Anxiety
- Irritability
- Depression
- Exhaustion
- Social withdrawal
- Trouble concentrating

According to the Alzheimer's Association, about 60 percent of Alzheimer's and dementia caregivers rate their stress levels as high or very high. And female caregivers are at the highest risk of suffering from the stress of caregiving.[1] This stress can affect not only your emotional well-being, but it can also undermine your relationship with your spouse, children, and other family members, especially those who share caregiving responsibilities with you.

Tension Among Caregivers

In the beginning stages of writing this book, I told a few people of this endeavor. One friend, in particular, listened to my family's story and really homed in on how we appeared to work so cooperatively with each other over an extended period of caregiving. To set the record straight, I've only known of one family who seemed to work cooperatively all of the time, who didn't make a decision for their loved one unless there was 100 percent consensus among family members, and where there appeared to be no friction or bitterness among family members.

This was not my family. But I can see where my friend might have gotten that impression. I didn't make it common practice to share with others the disagreements within my family, especially when they centered around how to best care for Mom.

Obviously, we all wanted what was best for Mom. But having four members in the immediate family meant there were many times when there was more than one belief about what was in her best interest. Sometimes we were able to work through our opposing opinions to come to a consensus. And sometimes we weren't. During those times, my sisters and I felt compelled to acquiesce to Dad's wishes. He was Mom's husband and her primary caregiver. And truthfully, none of us was eager to take over that role from Dad just to be able to make all the decisions single-handedly. In addition, there seemed to be an unspoken belief in my family that we needed to work as cooperatively as possible, whether we agreed all the time or not. Nonetheless, there were times when I firmly believed my opinion or belief was the best thing for Mom and it was very frustrating to yield to another point of view, especially one with which I didn't agree. I got through it by stewing in my own frustration until, ultimately, I was able to make peace with it or learn to live with it.

I know it's not that simple for some families, though. There are families that have experienced enormous turmoil and pain well before Alzheimer's disease came into the picture. Providing care for someone who might have caused you hurt in the past might leave you feeling angry and resentful. Or sharing caregiving with people you do not get along with could feel like an impossible task. Being an Alzheimer's caregiver can be challenging in the best of circumstances. Add the stress of strained family relationships, and it's just that much more challenging.

When to Get Help: Geriatric Care Managers

If you and your family are struggling with tension among caregivers, a **geriatric care manager** is a professional who might be able to offer your family guidance and support. Geriatric care managers are typically healthcare professionals with nursing, social work, gerontology, or mental health backgrounds. They perform an assessment and create a plan for your family moving forward, taking into account your family's specific challenges. Geriatric care managers work with families who want to do what is best for their loved one, but aren't sure what that is or how to proceed. In addition, if you have family members who live out of town or feel weighed down with other family, personal, or work responsibilities or family members who are in disagreement about how to care for their loved one, your family could benefit from the guidance of a geriatric care manager.

To locate a geriatric care manager in your area contact one of the following organizations:

- The National Association of Professional Geriatric Care Managers at www.aginglifecare.org
- The Area Agency on Aging Care at www.n4a.org/ eldercarelocator
- Community Resource Finder at www. communityresourcefinder.org

Strategies for Reducing Stress among Caregivers

There are many strategies to help families cope with the stress of caregiving. For one, listening to each other respectfully is so important. Alzheimer's disease progresses over many years, which means many decisions will need to be made regarding your loved one. Some decisions will be made quickly and easily with everyone in agreement, and others will be more complex, requiring ongoing discussions. Learning to listen respectfully enhances interactions that are positive, even when disagreements pop up between family members.

It's also important to discuss caregiving responsibilities and to keep the lines of communication open. Caregiving for your loved one requires both hands-on support and management of certain tasks, such as making doctor's appointments, grocery shopping, managing the finances, and driving (when your loved one stops driving) to name just a few. It's logical to assign duties, taking into account each caregiver's strengths. Your loved one's needs will likely change as time goes on because of the progressive nature of Alzheimer's disease. Likewise, caregivers' personal responsibilities might change over time, which means caregiving duties will need to be reviewed periodically to accommodate the caregivers' schedules and other considerations. In addition, keeping everyone up to date by meeting regularly (either in person or via conference call) to evaluate how things are going and to plan for the future should help support all members of the caregiving group.

While there are challenges and stressors when a family shares caregiving responsibilities, there are most certainly benefits as well. For one, the full responsibility does not fall on just one person. In my family, the caregiving duties were primarily divided among three people: Dad, my sister Mary, and me. My other sister, Barb, was supportive from a distance, as she lived out of town for the majority of the time we cared for Mom at home. When Barb moved back to Cincinnati, our caregiving circle became a foursome. Because Mom and Dad lived together, the primary caregiving responsibilities naturally fell on Dad. My sisters and I supported Dad on a regular basis by taking Mom to doctor appointments, giving her baths, driving her to and from adult day care (see below in this chapter), helping Dad with housekeeping duties, having Mom and Dad to our homes for dinner regularly, and staying with Mom so Dad could play an occasional round of golf. In addition, my sisters and I tended to be the ones to research any aspect of Mom's care or disease process that required information gathering (prospective doctors, day care centers, and eventually, nursing homes). We would then present our findings to Dad. As practical as it was to be providing care for Mom as a family unit, the emotional support cannot be overstated. We all experienced the unique grief associated with slowly losing someone to dementia. And during those times of both supporting my family and being supported by them, I was truly comforted in the knowledge that we understood each other's sadness and grief.

Long-Distance Caregiving

Whether you are your loved one's primary caregiver from afar or you're providing long-distance support to local caregivers, there are several steps you can take to be an involved and contributing member of your loved one's caregiving team.

- First and foremost, keep the lines of communication open among all members of the caregiving team, just as if you lived locally. Let them know you're interested in how they are managing their roles as caregivers and regularly ask them what you can do to help. (You can find resources available in your loved one's community through the Alzheimer's Association.)
- Whether or not you're the primary caregiver, have knowledge of your loved one's doctors, current medications and pharmacies, care providers, and neighbors.
- In addition, even if you're not the caregiver responsible for keeping track of and updating your loved one's fi-

nancial and legal documents and other personal papers, be aware of who is.

- During visits with your loved one, reassess the situation, as needs will change over time. Areas to assess include your loved one's hygiene, home and driving safety, and how your loved one is spending their time.
- Make sure your loved one is taking their medications as ordered.
- Check the pantry and refrigerator to evaluate if the food is appropriate and fresh.
- If possible, coordinate your loved one's doctor appointments for when you're in town and able to attend.
- Ask other caregivers, neighbors, and friends how they think your loved one is doing.
- While you might feel overwhelmed with duties during your visits, make time to spend quality time with your loved one.
- Finally, make every effort to give the primary caregiver a break from time to time by visiting when you can and taking over caregiving duties during visits.

Reducing Stress when Visiting the Doctor

Visiting the doctor can be a major source of stress for both you and your loved one. As ADEAR points out, "[a]dvance planning can help make the trip to the doctor's office go more smoothly."[2]

- Try to schedule the appointment for the person's best time of day. Also, ask the office staff what time of day the office is least crowded.
- Let the office staff know in advance that this person might be confused because of Alzheimer's disease. Ask them for help to make the visit go smoothly.

- Don't tell the person about the appointment until the day of the visit or even shortly before it's time to go. Be positive and matter-of-fact.
- Bring along something for the person to eat and drink and any materials or activities that he or she enjoys.
- Have a friend or another family member go with you on the trip, so that one of you can be with the person while the other speaks with the doctor.
- Take a brief summary listing the person's medical history, primary care doctor, and current medications.

Overcoming Isolation

Whether caregiving is shared with others or you are on your own, feelings of isolation are inevitable. The isolation that can come with Alzheimer's disease is a funny thing. I noticed it several years ago with my mom and dad. At the time I could find virtually nothing written on the subject to help me understand the reasons behind their isolation. But since then, I've read a few books that were written by caregivers and I noticed that they included stories of becoming increasingly isolated from family and friends who were not actively involved in their daily lives.

Knowing that others were experiencing the same isolation might have been comforting to me if it didn't leave me so unsettled. My dad is an intensely private person so over time, I was able to partly understand why some family and friends would fade away from my parents' lives. But only partly, because that still didn't answer why the question of why isolation seems to be such a common experience for both those with Alzheimer's disease and their caregivers.

Having now had years to ponder this problem, I've come up with a few explanations. First, caregivers often believe that they should be able to handle caregiving responsibilities without assistance from others. This leaves them deprived not only of the help of others but of their company as well. In addition, because many of the effects of dementia are considered socially unacceptable (including incontinence and other hygiene issues, trouble with communication, and unpredictable behavior, all of which are covered in earlier chapters), caregivers might also shy away from the company of others because they want to protect their loved one's dignity.

The person with Alzheimer's disease also might avoid social interaction to protect their own dignity. If they are having problems communicating with others, they might become quiet and withdrawn in social situations, or they might leave the room. And if they feel safer at home and uncomfortable in social settings away from home, they're unlikely to go out at all. This can increase not only their own feelings of isolation but their caregiver's as well.

To complicate matters, family and friends might pull away from you and your loved one. They might lack understanding about dementia and feel uncomfortable with its effects, especially communication difficulties and hygiene issues.

So what can you do to combat isolation, both your loved one's and your own?

Encourage Visitors

Invite family and friends to visit, and prepare them ahead of time for what to expect. Give them a heads up about unusual behaviors, communication difficulties, and hygiene issues they might encounter. Let them in on tactics that usually promote a positive interaction with your loved one and, conversely, the ones that provoke anxiety and agitation. In other words, suggest what they should or shouldn't try to do or say when they're with your loved one. It might also help to educate your family and friends about Alzheimer's disease and its effects by offering them reading materials and directing them to key websites.

Go out Together

You can also try to go out more with your loved one. Although it might require some advance thought and preparation, by continuing to participate in the activities you and your loved one enjoy for as long as possible, you'll both feel less isolated. But because these outings can also be a major source of caregiver stress, here are some suggestions for lessening the risk of stress if you do venture out together:

- Carry an extra set of clothes and undergarments with you whenever you leave the house for any length of time
- When away from home, locate the bathrooms in case your loved one needs to use one quickly
- If you plan to eat away from home, consider your loved one's special dietary needs and, if necessary, bring prepared foods they can eat without difficulty
- If your loved one has particular times of the day that are difficult, try to avoid activities away from home during those times

Finally, if your loved one does OK in a social setting for an hour, stay for only forty-five minutes and then go home. Don't push their limit or go beyond it. In our experience, the consequences of Mom being overwhelmed while out were entirely unpredictable. Sometimes she would calm down when she was back in the familiarity of her home, but sometimes she would remain anxious or agitated for the rest of the day. Be aware that your loved one's tolerance for most, if not all, things will decrease as the disease progresses. Even things that they really enjoyed in the past might upset them. Respect their limitations. Going out in public might create more problems than it's worth. Having pushed Mom to her limit or beyond more than once, I can truthfully say it was not worth the stress she experienced, and it was definitely not worth the avoidable stress we put on ourselves.

Join a Support Group

Finally, consider joining a caregiver support group. Support groups provide an opportunity to get out and meet others going through some of the same experiences. You can share stories, get helpful hints for coping, and even obtain information about treatment options and long-term care facilities. The Alzheimer's Association sponsors support groups in all fifty states. However, not everyone lives close to cities with Alzheimer's Association sponsored support groups. Local churches, senior centers, and your loved one's physician and office staff are good places to inquire about local caregiver support groups. If an online support group sounds more attractive to you, it doesn't matter where you live (as long as you have internet access). However, always verify with your loved one's physician any advice you receive online.

Reducing Stress

As mentioned above, the stress of being a caregiver cannot be overstated, but it also cannot and should not be ignored. Not only can stress take an emotional toll on you, it can undermine your physical health as well. Insomnia and sleep deprivation are common side effects of stress, as are frequent headaches, body aches, and weight gain. In addition to eating too much, stressed-out caregivers might drink or smoke too much. The stress of caregiving can also weaken your immune system, making you more susceptible to colds and flus, which can be passed on to your loved one.

If you're having any physical or emotional problems, I urge you to make your physician aware of them. If you don't take care of yourself, how can you take care of your loved one? The ramifications of your stress go beyond you. Caregivers under stress are more likely than others to make mistakes with their loved one's medications. What's more, not only might your loved one pick up your colds or flu, they might also pick up on some signs of your stress, which can only increase their feelings of inadequacy and even guilt. So de-stressing is not only good medicine for you, it's good for your loved one as well. And some of the best stress busters are also among the best things you can do to stay healthy ... and happy.

Exercise Regularly

There is considerable evidence that exercise can have a positive impact on caregiver (and other) stress. Indeed, regular exercise provides numerous benefits to your mind and body. Various brain chemicals are stimulated during exercise that could improve your mood, and energy is boosted as a result of oxygen and nutrients being delivered to your system. Exercise can also help you better manage a variety of health conditions, as well as reduce the risk of acquiring certain diseases such as type 2 diabetes, heart disease, stroke, and even some cancers. Whether you're looking to lose weight or maintain weight loss, exercise helps both.

You might think you don't have the time, energy, or desire to exercise regularly. But think of the benefits and look beyond push-ups, sit-ups, and chin-ups. Exercise doesn't have to be tedious or boring. Make it fun by choosing something you truly enjoy, such as dancing, bowling, or even gardening.

If you're a caregiver who already incorporates regular exercise into your life, keep it up! I'm sure you can vouch for its benefits. If not, how do you get started? How often should you exercise? How vigorous should your workout be? Well, as I'm not a doctor, it would be irresponsible of me to advise you on those particulars. So talk to your doctor. Knowing your health history, your doctor will be able to counsel you on the appropriate way to proceed with incorporating an exercise regimen into your life as well as advise you on other preventive health measures that can be challenging to caregivers, such as maintaining a healthy diet and getting adequate sleep. And speaking of sleep, if you do incorporate regular exercise into your life, you might notice an improvement in your sleep.

Get a Good Night's Sleep

As caregivers, there are many distractions to hinder our chances of getting the quality sleep we need. Our world can be loud, bright, fast paced, and stressful. Being a caregiver to someone with sleep disturbances adds another layer of stress. If your loved one is not sleeping through the night, chances are you are not either. Please do not underestimate your need for sleep. Sleep is vital to our well-being and its benefits are considerable.

Benefits of Sleep

Sleep can:
- Help you think more clearly
- Help you have quicker reflexes
- Help you focus better
- Be restorative

Conversely, lack of adequate sleep can:
- Interfere with your productivity at work
- Put you at higher risk for traffic accidents
- Negatively affect your mood
- Be detrimental to your health over time

Approaches to Improve Sleep

There are countless approaches (besides counting sheep) that can help you get a good night's sleep, including the following:

- Go to bed the same time each night and get up at the same time each morning
- Sleep in a dark, quiet, comfortable environment
- Exercise daily (but not right before bedtime)
- Limit the use of electronics before bedtime
- Relax before bedtime (a warm bath or reading might help)
- Avoid alcohol and stimulants such as caffeine and nicotine late in the day
- Take a break
- Consult a healthcare professional if you have ongoing sleep problems

One of the best ways to relieve stress is to take time out to do something you find fun or relaxing every day. Whether it's a massage, a manicure, yoga class, a bike ride, reading a novel, or just taking a walk, making time for the things you love to do truly is fuel that can sustain you through each day of caregiving. You might think this is impossible because of your caregiving responsibilities. But it's vitally important for you to continue to participate in activities you enjoy, even if that means entrusting your loved one's care to someone you trust while you're away. This is a good time to call on family and friends who have offered to help with your loved one.

Ask for and Accept Help

You deserve all the help you can get, be it someone to help you shoulder the responsibilities of caring for your loved one, a shoulder massage, or just a shoulder to cry on. If you reach out and ask for help, you are *not* being selfish. You are doing what's best for both you and your loved one.

I know that asking for help is easier said than done. If you're like me, it's so much easier to offer help than to accept it. But if you're blessed enough to have people in your life who you trust and who want to lighten your load, let them. Here's another way to think about this: If someone you cared about was going through a difficult time, would you want to help them get through it a bit more easily? How would you feel if you were denied the chance to help someone you cared about?

Asking for and accepting help is just the beginning. Actually getting the kind of help you need is not always as easy as you might think. I remember when Mom was really declining the last few months at home. Looking back, it was obvious that we needed help, but it wasn't nearly as clear then because we were focused entirely on just trying to get through each day. If asked, "Do you need help?" I think we would have answered with a yes, but I don't recall any of us having the foggiest idea of the type of assistance we needed. This appears to be a fairly common trait of Alzheimer's caregivers because there seem to be many caregivers attempting to care for their loved ones with little assistance. However, there is help out there.

Getting the Help You Need

Be it for a few hours or several days, taking an occasional break from caregiving is essential to your well-being. Whether or not your family and friends are able to pitch in, there are people and organizations that can help relieve you of some of the burdens of caregiving.

Home Healthcare Services

Getting part-time help is a great way to ease the burden and stress of caregiving. Home healthcare services can send a health aide to your loved one's home to help out or provide companionship for them for several hours or even overnight. Medicare might pay some of the costs, but you might be responsible for most.

The services provided by a home health agency or an independent homecare provider are extensive and varied. Below are several different types of home healthcare providers and the services they provide:

- **Skilled healthcare professionals** include nurses, physical therapists, occupational therapists, and speech therapists. Depending on their training, they might be able to perform many health-related tasks, such as changing bandages and dressings and assisting with medication administration. They might also offer various types of therapy such as physical, occupational, and speech.
- **Licensed health professionals** can give injections and provide other medical services.
- **Home health aides** are usually trained and state-certified when they work for an agency. They can help with bathing, dressing, transferring, toileting, and eating. However, they might also be able to help with needed tasks more commonly associated with a homemaker or companion such as cooking, shopping, and laundry.
- **Homemakers** or **companions** can help with light housekeeping, meal preparation, transportation, and companionship. They are not trained to provide hands-on assistance with activities of daily living such as bathing and dressing.

Keep in mind that not all states require licensing for home healthcare providers. If you choose a provider who is employed by a company or agency, they likely had a background or reference check prior to being hired. However, don't make that assumption—ask instead. And be sure to get and check references. (In Chapter 9: Getting the Best Care for Your Loved One, I'll provide more information on how to evaluate home healthcare services.)

Meal Services

Having someone else occasionally prepare meals can be a godsend. While it's great if friends and relatives are able to pitch in with meals, meal services are a wonderful option. They can save you time (fewer trips to the grocery store and time spent preparing meals) and even money (the cost can vary from free to a small fee). One of the best resources is Meals on Wheels (www.mealsonwheelsamerica.org/). Meals on Wheels is the oldest and largest national meal service and has over 5,000 community-based senior nutrition and other services that are provided by more than two million volunteers. The cost varies depending on location and financial need.

Respite Care

The word *respite* refers to taking a break from the challenges and burdens of caregiving. Homecare services, meal services, and adult day care (see below) are all examples of respite that provide care from as little as an hour to several hours a day. However, there might be times when a longer respite period is necessary. This type of respite care provides short-term, full-time care for a loved one at home or in a healthcare facility, usually for up to five days. This allows a caregiver to go on a short vacation, deal with business or other personal issues, or just get a break from caregiving.

Many agencies that provide home healthcare services also provide home respite services to accommodate extended caregiving needs as well. That's really a positive if you and your loved one are familiar with a particular agency and the care providers they employ. Some assisted living facilities, nursing homes, and hospitals offer respite for overnight, weekend, or extended stays as well. In some cases, Medicare might cover the cost for up to five days in a row in an inpatient facility. To find out more about respite services, including what's available in your area, contact the ARCH National Respite Network and Resource Center (www.archrespite.org).

Adult Day Care

Another option that can give you a break from daytime caregiving responsibilities is having your loved one attend an adult day care program. This can be a huge benefit not only for caregivers but for their loved ones as well. Adult day care can provide opportunities for socialization in a safe and secure environment while also giving structure to your loved one's day.

On more than one occasion, the counselor from the Alzheimer's Association spoke to me about the benefits of adult day care for both Mom and Dad. For Dad, it would provide respite from the demands of full-time caregiving. For Mom, it would provide structure in a social setting that offered a variety of activities for those with cognitive impairment and dementia. Most importantly, though, the counselor said that Mom could start becoming comfortable receiving care from people outside our family. Of all the valuable counseling and advice I received through the years, this was one concept that stuck with me as being one of the most helpful.

But implementing that advice wasn't easy. Knowing the progressive nature of Alzheimer's disease, I was aware that there might come a time when our family could no longer care for Mom at home and that she might ultimately need to be placed in a full-time care facility. And as I was much more comfortable dealing pragmatically with Mom's needs, the counselor's reasoning that an adult day care program would be a good intermediary step made a lot of sense to me. Although I was sold on the concept of adult day care immediately, it was a struggle to convince my dad that the positive outweighed the negative. The negative, according to Dad, was that Mom would never accept or adjust to adult day care. Nevertheless, his staunch opinion didn't stop my sisters and me from reintroducing the idea of adult day care from time to time, unfortunately to no avail. So eventually, assuming it was a dead issue, we stopped talking about it and the status quo continued.

A few years later, Mom was evaluated by a dementia neurologist. One of his recommendations was for her to attend adult day care. The reasons he cited were very similar to what I had heard from the Alzheimer's Association counselor several years before. Our dead issue was resurrected. With a physician recommending adult day care, Dad agreed to it, albeit unenthusiastically. When Mary called to let me know that Mom's new doctor had recommended adult day care, she said: "Now we can put to use all the information you've been gathering on adult day care centers." It's true that I had researched adult day care centers in Cincinnati. It's also true, in a dramatic show of frustration, that I had tossed all that information some time before after another unsuccessful conversation with Dad on the subject. I really cursed that impetuous stunt, knowing that I had to start researching again from scratch.

When we compared the activities an appropriate adult day center could consistently provide to what a typical day currently looked like for Mom, my family and I were able to get to a place of resignation, if not universal acceptance. As it turns out, Dad's concerns were unwarranted: Mom did accept and adjust to adult day care. Dad got respite when Mom attended adult day care a couple of days each week, and he even began counting on it when he was planning a golf game with family and friends. We were also lucky that the center we chose was a good fit for Mom.

Conclusion

In the next chapter you'll find detailed information and advice about choosing an appropriate adult day care center and other services for your loved one. And because at some point, they might need more help than you and your family or a day care program can provide, I'll also include information on how to find the best long-term care for your loved one.

Resources

General Information on Being a Caregiver

▶ **ADEAR (The Alzheimer's Disease Education and Referral Center)**
Detailed information on caring for yourself as an Alzheimer's caregiver: www.nia.nih.gov/alzheimers/publication/caring-yourself
An extensive list of published works and resources provides advice and support for caregivers: www.nia.nih.gov/alzheimers/relieving-stress-anxiety-resources-alzheimers-caregivers

▶ **Family Caregiver Alliance**
Issues relevant to caregivers ("Caregiving and Controlling Frustration," "Holding a Family Meeting," "Caregiving with Your Siblings," "Emotional Side of Caregiving," "Taking Care of You: Self-Care for Family Caregivers," and "Caregiving and Ambiguous Loss") are presented in a fact- and tip-sheet format. Also access the "Handbook for Long-Distance Caregivers."
www.caregiver.org/fact-sheets
www.caregiver.org/sites/caregiver.org/files/pdfs/op_2003_long_distance_handbook.pdf

▶ **The American Association of Retired Persons: The Caregiving Resource Center**
"Care for Yourself" has pertinent articles focused on caregiver needs, such as managing the stress of being a caregiver, paying attention to your own health, and finding the support you need with caregiving.
www.aarp.org/home-family/caregiving/?intcmp=GLBNAV-SL-HEA-CARE

▶ **The Mayo Clinic**
"Alzheimer's: Dealing with Family Conflict"
www.mayoclinic.org/healthy-lifestyle/caregivers/in-depth/alzheimers/art-20047365

▶ *The Alzheimer's Project* (video)
HBO's *The Alzheimer's Project* presents a series of videos on many aspects of Alzheimer's disease of interest to family and caregivers.
www.hbo.com/alzheimers/index.html

▶ *The Forgetting: A Portrait of Alzheimer's* (video)
PBS's Emmy award-winning documentary based on the best-selling book by David Shenk.
www.pbs.org/program/forgetting/

▶ **Peter Rabins Alzheimer's Family Support Center**
"Caregiver Guilt—Memory and Alzheimer's Disease" (video)
www.youtube.com/watch?v=15-s68-hngk&feature=youtu.be

Support Groups

▶ **The Alzheimer's Association** 1–800–272–3900
The Alzheimer's Association online Caregiver Center addresses such issues as day-to-day, hands-on caregiving issues and caregiver health, as well as providing online support through message boards and ALZConnected, the Alzheimer's Association's online support community. Local support groups are listed as well.
www.alz.org/care/alzheimers-dementia-support-help.asp

▶ **Community Resource Finder**
The Community Resource Finder through the
Alzheimer's Association allows you to access listings of
support groups in your area.
www.communityresourcefinder.org/

▶ **The American Association of Retired Persons:**
The Caregiving Resource Center
Join monthly "Chat with an Expert" online meetings
hosted by AARP's Caregiver Advisory Panel, made up
of experts in the fields of aging, caregiving, psychiatry,
nutrition, and more. Monthly chats cover a wide range
of topics that affect all types of caregivers. Some are
directly related to Alzheimer's disease and caregiving
issues unique to caring for a loved one with dementia.
And many others are focused on family dynamics and
challenges. AARP's online community connects you to
other caregivers.
www.aarp.org/home-family/
caregiving/?intcmp=GLBNAV-SL-HEA-CARE

Help with Travel

▶ **TSA Cares (through the Transportation Security**
Administration)
1–855–787–2227
"TSA Cares is a helpline to assist travelers with
disabilities and medical conditions. TSA recommends
that passengers call 72 hours ahead of travel for
information about what to expect during screening....
TSA Cares will serve as an additional, dedicated
resource specifically for passengers with disabilities,
medical conditions or other circumstances or for their
loved ones who want to prepare for the screening
process prior to flying."

Whatever your mode of transport, the sooner you notify the company you're using for transportation, the better they can prepare for your needs. www.tsa.gov/travel/passenger-support

Finding a Geriatric Care Manager

▶ **The National Association of Professional Geriatric Care Managers**
Access listings of geriatric care managers in your area. caremanager.org

Nine

Getting the Best Care for Your Loved One

The previous chapter on caregiver survival demonstrated that getting outside help is exceptionally important not only for you and your family, but for your loved one as well. However, deciding what kind of help is best and taking the plunge to get it is easier said than done.

Adult Day Care

As described in the last chapter, our family debated the issue of adult day care for Mom for many years before finally deciding to find a day program that would be appropriate for her. Once we made that decision, we started researching the various options. In the course of doing that research, we found that there are three different types of adult day care centers: social, medical/health, and specialized.

Even though some health-related services are provided at a social day program, they are limited. The focus is primarily on recreation. Usually, meals or snacks are provided as well. In general, the difference between a social and a medical/health day program is in the level of healthcare provided. In addition to meals and social activities, more intensive health and therapeutic services are provided in a medical/health day program. The center we chose for Mom was considered a medical/ health day center. Although she didn't require the level of care they provided from a medical standpoint, the center was conveniently located and had a lot of social activities, which were priorities for us.

As the name implies, specialized day programs are limited to providing services to specific populations, such as people with Alzheimer's disease or other dementias. They might or might not be able to manage the additional needs that a medical/health day program manages, such as blood pressure monitoring and medication administration. If you're not sure, ask what specific medical services they provide when you visit the center.

Regardless of the type, most adult day care centers offer a variety of nonmedical services including social activities, door-to-door transportation service, meals, personal care, and therapeutic activities. Although the day program my mom attended provided door-to-door transportation, the consensus in my family was that, with Mom's high level of dementia, it was more appropriate for us drive her to and from the center. Maybe we didn't give Mom enough credit that she could handle being driven by someone other than us, but we just didn't think she would tolerate the drive to and from the center in an unfamiliar van with an unfamiliar driver.

At Mom's day program, they regularly offered arts and crafts, and once or twice a month, an Alzheimer's Association staff member would lead an art program for the clients with Alzheimer's disease or other dementias. In addition, the center celebrated holidays by throwing parties. A couple of times each month they also offered outings to local restaurants for lunch. However, those outings were limited to those who were able to travel in a bus that had steps and dine in a restaurant with minimal assistance. For those who couldn't participate, lunch on those days would be delivered to the center from local eateries. Regardless of whether field trips were scheduled, breakfast and lunch were a daily service. There was even a section in the dining room for clients who required help eating. While Mom never required that level of care, I appreciated that it was offered for those individuals who did. Without that level of service, many people would not be able go to that center.

Personal care was also provided, and the center requested that families provide a change of clothes should a client's clothing become wet or soiled. It was commonplace for staff to assist clients with toileting. Social activities included bingo and other games, Bible study, and movies. Gentle exercise was offered on a regular basis both for those who could walk on their own and for those restricted to wheelchairs. For special occasions, live music was provided by local musicians.

Healthcare professionals at many day programs are able to monitor various aspects of their clients' health such as weight, blood pressure, and diabetes. In addition, the nursing staff can help with medication management and administration. Rehabilitation therapy is also commonly offered. My mom's center provided all of these health services. Had we chosen a social adult day center, most of these services wouldn't have been available to her.

While making the decision about what type of care to choose might seem overwhelming at first, the National Adult Day Services Association (NADSA) is an excellent resource that can help you navigate a type of care that might be completely new to you (www.nadsa.org).

How to Choose an Adult Day Care Center

There are many things to consider when looking for an adult day care center. For example, because not all states license and regulate adult day care centers, from center to center there might be major differences, such as client-to-staff ratio and variety of services offered. Ultimately, it will be your responsibility to educate yourself about the centers you are considering for your loved one. NADSA has a page with a state-by-state list of regulations and associations. This is a good place to start your research: www.nadsa.org/providers/state-regulations/.

The first thing to do (unless you already have a day program in mind) is to compile a list of centers you might consider. You can find them by word of mouth or through local agencies on aging. Your loved one's doctor or other healthcare providers might also have good suggestions. Finally, the following organizations offer online tools to help you find day programs and other types of respite services in your area:

- The National Adult Day Services Association (www. nadsa.org)
- The Alzheimer's Association (www. communityresourcefinder.org)
- US Administration on Aging's Eldercare Locator (www. eldercare.gov)
- The ARCH National Respite Network and Resource Center (www.archrespite.org)

Once you've narrowed down your list of potential day programs, you'll want to find out as much as you can about each center you are considering. Although each family will have its own criteria and issues they regard as important, the Alzheimer's Association recommends asking the following questions of each center you visit:[i]

- What are the hours, fees, and services? (Be sure to ask about the minimum attendance requirements and the notification policy for absences.)
- What types of programs are offered?
- Are people with dementia separated from other participants or included in general activities?

- Will the center evaluate the person's needs? How will this evaluation be accomplished? How often will it be repeated?
- Is staff trained in dementia issues?
- What types of healthcare professionals are on staff? How do you screen them?
- How are emergency situations handled?
- How do you ensure the safety of the participants?
- Is transportation available?

It's also a good idea to take notes so you can later compare facilities based on the answers you've gotten. When you visit a center, talk to various staff and observe their interactions with clients. Also, try to talk to family members whose loved ones attend the center to help determine how appropriate it might be for your loved one.

When you do tour prospective adult day centers, be prepared. My sister Barb and I toured the adult day care center Mom ultimately attended and spoke to its director before deciding upon it. Knowing the population they serve, we should not have been surprised by what we observed. But we were. The clients we observed looked different than those in a senior center that serves a mainly self-sufficient clientele, which I think is what we expected. The folks who attend a day program might have dementia, developmental delays, or other health conditions. They might require help with feeding, toileting, taking medication, or receiving medical treatments. They might walk independently or need a cane, walker, or wheelchair. A good adult day center has staff who are trained to care for all of those needs.

Homecare and Home Healthcare

While some people choose to get either homecare or home healthcare for their loved ones before considering adult day care, we didn't consider it until adult day care was no longer working for Mom. She had stopped going to the center because of the onset of some challenging behaviors, especially agitation. It was becoming more and more difficult for the staff to intervene and to redirect Mom when she became agitated. In other words, once she was agitated, she generally stayed agitated until we picked her up for the day.

When Mom stopped going to adult day care, Dad was deprived of the part-time respite he really needed. Mom's sundowning as well emotional behaviors, such as confusion, agitation, anger, and pacing more often than not continued throughout the entire night. This made it extremely hard for Dad to care for her. As I mentioned in previous chapters, if a loved one is not sleeping through the night, chances are neither is the caregiver, so we were very concerned about Dad. Although Mary and I helped as much as possible with caregiving duties, we were unable to be there all the time because we both had our own families to tend to.

Mom was finally introduced to home healthcare during a period of upheaval for both of my parents. Dad had spent the better part of two weeks away from home due to consecutive hospitalizations to treat an abnormal heart rhythm. During his time away from home, my sisters and I took shifts staying with Mom. She had always been comfortable with Mary and me as caregivers. However, Barb had lived in Los Angeles before Mom was diagnosed with even mild cognitive impairment and thus Mom was not accustomed to Barb being her caregiver. Although Barb jumped in wholeheartedly to help anyway, sadly, Mom was not as comfortable with her as she was with Mary and me. Additionally, not having Dad's calm and consistent presence in her life for that period of time took a big toll on her, and she worsened considerably while Dad was away from home.

To minimize Dad's stress following his hospitalizations, my sisters and I decided it would be beneficial for him to recover at one of our houses for a week before returning home to care for Mom. By then, Mom was requiring a lot more care than before as well as almost constant supervision.

Given the circumstances, it didn't take much convincing to get Dad's OK to begin part-time home healthcare for Mom. And considering Dad's steadfast refusal of help outside our family, this was a huge accomplishment. While his heart had returned to beating as it should, Dad was run down and exhausted from his recent health scare and hospitalizations. We also started noticing the tiniest of cracks in his previously impenetrable armor of patience. Truthfully, my dad's ability to maintain composure and patience with Mom over the previous several years left me amazed. But now Mary, Barb and I most definitely needed to keep an eye on him and how he was coping with his own recovery as well as his return to the role of caregiver.

With the benefit of hindsight, I realize a few key things. First, home healthcare was absolutely necessary during that time for several reasons: Mom needed constant supervision and Dad needed a lot of help taking care of Mom. That being said, it was a terrible time to introduce Mom to home healthcare for the same reasons homecare became necessary. She was very unsettled and her dementia was worsening. It was becoming more difficult to communicate successfully with her because she was so confused. Mom couldn't understand what we were attempting to convey to her, and we were having a more difficult time figuring out what she wanted or needed. As a result, she responded by becoming angry and agitated. That pattern became the norm for us the last few months she was at home.

Expecting Mom to accept and be comfortable with an unfamiliar caregiver at that time was unrealistic. But when

Dad, Mary, or I couldn't be there, Mom needed to have a home health aide to stay with her and keep her safe. Some days it worked smoothly (like when she had slept the night before) and others it didn't. On those occasions, Mom was confused, agitated, and angry. More often than not, I bet Mom was a tough assignment for her aide. I do not share this story to discourage you from enlisting the help that home healthcare can provide for you and your loved one. I share it in the hope that you will consider home healthcare before a crisis occurs.

Assessing Your Homecare Needs

To help you decide if you need homecare for your loved one, the Alzheimer's Association suggests you take the following into consideration:[2]

- ❏ **Safety:** Is it safe for your loved one to be home alone? Do they require 24-hour supervision or care, or supervision for some activities such as cooking? (See Chapter 6: Safety First.)
- ❏ **Health:** Does your loved one require specialized healthcare at home, such as help with medications, dressing changes, or blood sugar monitoring?
- ❏ **Routine Care:** Does your loved one need more care than you or your family can provide for toileting, bathing, or other hygiene-related issues? Is caring for them becoming difficult for you (or another major caregiver) to handle physically, emotionally, or time-wise?

Checking Credentials

According to the National Institute on Aging (NIA), some healthcare services and their home aides are very good, while unfortunately others are not. Therefore, NIA recommends that you carefully check out the agencies before signing an agreement. Medicare's online tool for comparing agencies is an excellent place to start: www.medicare.gov/homehealthcompare/search.html. (You can also call Medicare for information about specific home healthcare agencies). Pay special attention to the quality-of-care star ratings and patient survey results. You should also check to see if the agency you're considering has any complaints filed against them. This information should be available through the Better Business Bureau as well as your local community, county, or state agencies. Finally, be sure to get personal references from several people who have used the service or provider you're considering using.

It's also important to make sure the agency is licensed if your state requires it. Not all states require homecare and home healthcare agencies to be licensed and reviewed regularly. However, all Medicare-certified agencies are required to comply with federal regulations. To illustrate, there is no state licensure for home health agencies in my home state of Ohio, but all direct-care workers must undergo a criminal background check prior to employment at a home health agency in Ohio. To check on your state's licensure and other regulatory requirements, contact your state's department of health or your local agency on aging (which can also help you find a homecare agency in your area).

The following resources can be helpful in checking credentials for any home healthcare agencies you are considering:

- The National Adult Day Services Association (www.nadsa.org)
- The Alzheimer's Association (www.communityresourcefinder.org)
- US Administration on Aging's Eldercare Locator (www.eldercare.gov)
- The ARCH National Respite Network and Resource Center (www.archrespite.org)
- Medicare (www.medicare.gov/homehealthcompare/search.html)

How to Evaluate Home Healthcare Services and Providers

As with evaluating adult day care centers, there are important questions you should ask when evaluating home services:[3]

- **Services needed:** Does the homecare provider offer specific services for people with dementia?
- **Patient Care plans:** How are care plans created and reviewed? Ideally, your family and loved one (if able) should be involved.
- **Training and experience:** Do staff have training or experience in working with someone with dementia? Are those credentials verified? In other words, can the agency provide you with documentation that confirms their care providers have training and/or experience in caring for those with dementia?
- **Background check:** Does the agency, service provider, or homecare facility conduct background checks on all staff?
- **Backups:** What is the procedure if the homecare provider is sick, on vacation, or quits?
- **References:** Ask the care provider for at least three references. Contact the families and ask about their experience with the provider, the care their loved one received, and any concerns or problems the family had.
- **On-site visits:** Ask if the care provider can come to your home to meet you and your loved one. Does the care provider interact and communicate well with your loved one?

When Homecare Is Not Enough

In my experience, unless you're living in the same home as the person with Alzheimer's disease, you don't really know what's going on twenty-four hours a day. While Dad was Mom's primary caregiver and the person she most depended on, Mary and I were participating in her care and offering respite to Dad several days per week. That being said, we were not there regularly enough as evening wore on when her symptoms of sundowning worsened, and we were not there overnight to either witness what was going on or to help out.

At one point, I attended a lecture given by a respected physician in the fields of geriatrics and Alzheimer's disease. The talk was informal and was focused on practical day-to-day caregiver concerns. He allowed for audience questions during his talk and, as you can imagine, there were many. About midway through the evening, the topic turned to nursing homes.

There are many difficult issues to face for both the person with Alzheimer's disease and their caregivers, and making the decision to place your loved one in a full-time care facility is certainly one of the most difficult. The physician told the audience that putting your loved one in a nursing home is often times harder on the family and caregivers than it is on the patient. At the time, though, I could only imagine the effect it would have on my mom.

Through the years, as Mom's dementia advanced, my family and I discussed the possibility of ultimately needing to place her in a nursing home. During these family discussions, where Mary and Dad expressed their thoughts and feelings of sadness, I spoke (and thought) matter-of-factly about the probability of Mom needing that level of care if she lived long enough for the disease to progress to its later stages. It's not that I wouldn't let myself feel the emotions that Mary and Dad expressed during these discussions; rather, my emotions were buried so deeply that I was completely unaware of their existence. Boy, was I living in a fool's paradise!

Mom's dementia got considerably worse when Dad started dealing with his own health issues. Who knows if the disease was going to progress the way it did on its own, or if Dad being diagnosed with a health condition that required time away from her nudged it along a little bit?

The three months after Dad's hospitalization brought more stress and uncertainty than we had faced in all the years Mom had been living with dementia. She stopped attending adult day care, and Dad finally admitted that Mom had begun lashing out at him physically. This was a huge change for Dad to admit that things were not going well at home and a huge change in Mom behaviorally speaking. She had never been physically aggressive. In addition, it was at about this time that we added homecare services to assist us in caring for Mom at home.

All the while we were in close contact with Mom's doctor. First, to rule out a physical cause for her behavior changes (pain or a possible infection or illness); and second, to begin the tedious process of adjusting or changing some of her medications. Mom's symptoms of restlessness, agitation, sleeplessness, and generalized surliness waxed and waned during this period. After a rare night of sleep, her attitude and behavior were remarkably improved. However, those days (and nights) became less frequent with each passing week, with her sundowning symptoms appearing earlier almost each passing day. And still we clung to the belief that if we could get Mom on the right medication regimen, her hard-to-manage behaviors might become manageable again.

The one bright spot during this period was that this all happened when my sister Barb moved back to Cincinnati. We were not only thrilled to have all three sisters back in the same city, we also really needed the extra help Barb could provide.

We were anxiously awaiting the end of the Christmas holidays when Mom was scheduled to be evaluated by a geriatric psychiatrist recommended by her physician. One morning, I got a call from Mary informing me that Dad had called her in the middle of the night to ask for her help with Mom. Mom had never gone to sleep that night and was extremely agitated. Looking for guidance, I called her doctor, who luckily was available by phone. He said that Mom needed to be admitted to the hospital through the emergency room. This would also be the quickest way she could be evaluated by that geriatric psychiatrist, as he ran the unit where she would be admitted. As difficult as it was leaving Mom in the hospital that first evening (and every evening for that matter), there was comfort in knowing that she was in the right place and relief that our responsibility for caregiving was on hold, at least for the time being.

After visiting Mom one evening early in her hospitalization, which was to last nearly three weeks, Dad, Barb, and I walked out of the unit with one of Mom's nurses. As we were about to say goodnight, the nurse asked us if we had started looking for a nursing home. Caught completely off guard, we looked at each other and then proceeded awkwardly, trying to convince her that all Mom really needed was to get her medications adjusted. We explained that the last three months had been extremely hard on her because her routine had been seriously disrupted by Dad's health problems. She gently persisted and so did we. But at some point, everyone got quiet.

I had spent many years discussing this possibility with my family in a practical and emotionless way, and I thought I was being strong and realistic. But I'm being completely honest when I tell you that this was the first time I felt the sadness and heartbreak from facing the truth that Mom could no longer live at home. It hit me like a ton of bricks, and I wept in the nurse's arms.

My sisters, Dad, and I talked frequently over the next few days about next steps, and we were not always in agreement. But, by this time, Mom's doctor was urging us to start searching for an appropriate nursing home for her. So we did.

We learned a lot through the process of finding the *right* nursing home for Mom. But we learned the most from making an unwise choice the first time around. Our main criterion for choosing Mom's first nursing home was location. My family and I lived within a fifteen-minute drive from each other's homes, and at the time, it was important for the location to be convenient for all of us as we knew we'd be visiting Mom frequently. The first nursing home we chose also had a secure unit (where the doors leading out of the unit were secured or locked) where the dementia residents were housed. That was essential because we had a hunch Mom would wander and pace back and forth if given the opportunity, and she needed a safe, secure space to do that.

What we didn't notice during the tour was that Mom would have been one of the few residents who could wander and pace, because she and a couple of other residents were the only ones able to walk independently. We also didn't notice that, while it was a secure unit, there were many residents living there without dementia. Having people with dementia living in the same unit as those without dementia is not in the best interest of either group for several reasons. Residents who are alert and oriented should not have to tolerate residents who might be prone to rummaging and other common dementia behaviors such as wandering in and out of their rooms any time. Just as importantly, though, residents with dementia should be free to interact with each other and have the liberty to move about, either independently or with the help of walkers and wheelchairs if necessary. In the real world you will find folks with dementia living in the same units as those without dementia. In those instances, ask the long-term care facility's personnel how they manage their varied resident population so that all are living harmoniously.

Lastly, we wrongly assumed that all the residents would have dementia because it was a secure unit, something patients without dementia wouldn't necessarily need or want. Furthermore, we never thought to ask if it was acceptable for residents to wander in and out of each other's rooms because, quite truthfully, we didn't know to ask. It wasn't until Mom was admitted to that unit that we came to realize the wandering and pacing so many folks with Alzheimer's disease do was not considered acceptable by staff. Mom found herself in trouble with the staff almost every day for behaving like a person with dementia, which, of course, she was!

Lessons Learned

I'd like to share with you what we learned from that unfortunate experience. Just as I mentioned above that implementing home healthcare was less than ideal because we did so as a response to a crisis, choosing a nursing home in the middle of a crisis turned out to be no better. However, the upside to that first experience was that we had a much better idea of what we did and didn't want for Mom's next nursing home.

There can be huge differences from nursing home to nursing home. As an example, Mom's first nursing home and the one in which she now resides are both Medicare- and Medicaid-certified nursing homes, and both had earned a four-star (out of five stars) rating from Medicare. The ratings are the results of nursing home health inspections, quality measures, and staffing evaluations. Although both of the nursing homes had an above-average rating, we found major differences between the two facilities, primarily the culture and the philosophy of care, neither of which can be quantified in a rating system.

We also learned the following:
- There is no perfect nursing home, but there *are* very good ones.
- While a particular nursing home might be a wonderful fit for one person, it could be a poor fit for another. As

caregivers, we all evaluate nursing homes based on very personal feelings and priorities.

- Don't judge a book by its cover. Look past the shiny body of the facility to get to its heart, the patient care staff.
- No residential care facility can stop the progression of this disease. But the good news is that if a facility is able to manage a loved one's dementia-related behaviors well, they might actually seem improved compared to when they were living at home. That was the case with Mom.

I've had conversations with many caregivers who also experienced moving their loved ones from their first nursing home to another. At first, I was surprised by the number of people whose stories were similar to ours. That is, feeling forced to make that all-important decision as a reaction to a crisis either they or their loved one were experiencing. Also, not having thought through what qualities would be most desirable when evaluating prospective nursing homes given the particular challenges of their loved one's dementia. Then I started wondering if it was more than a coincidence that so many people with Alzheimer's disease had more than one nursing home experience—that the first nursing home they were admitted to was not the one in which they now reside.

When we decided to look for a new nursing home, we drew upon our first experience to help us make a much more informed choice. We decided location would still be considered, but it would not be the most important quality. In addition, our search focused on care facilities that had secure units where *all* of the residents had dementia. We felt that those facilities might have a different way of managing residents as they would all likely exhibit one or more dementia-related behaviors. We were hoping there were places that could manage these dementia-related behaviors, while still maintaining order and keeping the residents safe. Keeping Mom up and mobile was very important to us as well. We believed and continue to believe that being mobile tremendously impacts her quality of life. In addition, we asked questions about the staff who would be providing hands-on care for Mom. For example we asked about patient-to-staff ratio, but also whether care providers were specifically trained and experienced in dementia caregiving. We learned from our first experience that we were really interested in a place that embraced a more holistic style of resident management. In other words, we came to the task much better prepared than we had the first time.

Choose the Right Type of Facility

It wasn't until Mom was settled in her present nursing home that I started looking at the process we used to choose both nursing homes for Mom. I developed the following guide in hindsight, with the goal of helping others through the stressful process of choosing a residential care facility. First, it's helpful to understand the different types of residential facilities available to someone with Alzheimer's disease as detailed by the Alzheimer's Association:[4]

- **Retirement homes:** These homes are only appropriate for people with early-stage Alzheimer's disease who are still able to care for themselves independently.
- **Continuing care retirement communities:** These facilities provide different levels of care (independent living, assisted living, and nursing homecare) based on individual needs. In other words, a person can start out living there when they are completely independent, but as their needs change, different levels of care are provided (sometimes in different buildings) without having to move to a totally different facility.

- **Assisted living facilities:** These facilities bridge the gap between independent living and the need for full-time care in a nursing home.
- **Nursing homes:** Nursing homes provide 24/7 care and long-term medical treatment.
- **Alzheimer's specialty care units:** These are units within nursing homes or other healthcare facilities that are limited to caring for those with Alzheimer's disease and other dementias.

Create a Profile

Once you've decided on the type of facility you think would be the best fit, create a detailed profile of your loved one. This allows you to have in writing a current assessment of your loved one's status including key medical information and other major issues before you even visit a potential facility. Why is this important? Accurate and pertinent information about your loved one is just as important for you to share as it is for a prospective nursing home to receive. You're both deciding if a good fit is possible. It might be helpful to complete this profile with other involved family members, caregivers, or physicians.

Sample Profile

1. **Level of care needed:**
   - ❏ Toileting (independent   cuing   needs assistance total care)
   - ❏ Bathing (independent   cuing   needs assistance total care)
   - ❏ Brushing teeth (independent   cuing   needs assistance   total care)
   - ❏ Dressing (independent   cuing   needs assistance total care)
   - ❏ Eating (independent   cuing   needs assistance total care)

2. **Walking ability:**
   - ❏ Walks independently (steady gait   unsteady gait)
   - ❏ Walks with assistance (cane   walker)
   - ❏ Wheelchair dependent

3. **Behavior issues:**
   - ❏ Wandering (never   occasionally   frequently)
   - ❏ Hoarding/rummaging (never   occasionally frequently)
   - ❏ Sundowning (never   occasionally   frequently)
   - ❏ Physically aggressive behaviors (never   occasionally frequently)
   - ❏ Sexually explicit talk or behavior (never occasionally   frequently)

4. **Communication issues** (list barriers to and helpful hints for effective communication)

5. **Morning routine** (describe waking, dressing, toileting, and other hygiene issues)

6. **Evening and bedtime routine** (describe bathing, toileting, sleep, and other hygiene issues)

7. **Emotional issues** (describe mood and temperament changes in a typical day and night)

8. **Social issues** (describe interactions with other people one-on-one and in group settings)

9. **Favorite activities** (list)

10. **Medications** (list current medications and any allergies or reactions to them; how meds are taken, any difficulty swallowing, etc.)

11. **Other medical conditions or healthcare needs** (describe how they're being treated and by whom)

The above profile should help you keep in mind important issues and priorities as well as help you formulate key questions when you start investigating individual nursing or other residential homes. Had we done this, I think we would have been in a position to choose a more appropriate nursing home for Mom the first time around.

List Priorities and Considerations

Listing your major priorities and considerations will help clarify which features are most important to you in a prospective nursing home. Location, for example, is often a serious consideration. Is the location convenient enough for all members of the family to visit as often as they would like? Are there elderly or disabled family members who would like to visit? If they drive, can they safely drive to the nursing home as often as they would like? If they don't drive, are there other family members who can commit to regularly getting them to the nursing home to visit?

Another key issue for many families is whether the nursing home is a Medicare- or Medicaid-approved facility, meaning it accepts patients who are unable to pay for their care. A nursing home can cost about $100,000 per year. If you're able to pay out of pocket, at least initially, will you require a Medicare- or Medicaid-approved facility in the future?

You can usually get the above and other key information from the facility's website. www.medicare.gov is another good source of information. Health inspections, staffing, and quality measures are evaluated for each facility and a star value is awarded based on the results of the evaluation. If you still have unanswered questions, call the nursing home directly.

Consider Other Screening Questions

About Your Loved One

Below are some questions about other key issues that might help you decide if you want to proceed with a tour of the facility (you might want to add other questions based on your loved one's profile and your priorities):

- Do they take people with Alzheimer's disease?
- Are the residents with Alzheimer's disease housed in a secured or locked unit?
- If yes, is the unit dedicated to dementia patients exclusively?
- If not, are the residents with Alzheimer's disease housed with the general population?

About the Nursing Home Staff

- What is the staff-to-patient ratio during the day?
- Does the ratio change on evening shift, overnight, weekends, and holidays?
- Which medical professionals will be overseeing and managing your loved one's care? Physicians, physician assistants, nurse practitioners?
- What is the average length of service for the nursing home staff?
- Do they have experience dealing with dementia?
- Is there ongoing dementia-related training and education for staff who work in the dementia unit?
- If there are state-mandated minimum staff-to-patient ratios, how does the nursing home meet that requirement during staff illness, vacations, etc.?
- If substitute or temporary staff are used, are they nursing home employees, agency employees, or both?
- Knowing that caring for the dementia population is very stressful, what plan, if any, do they have in place to decrease staff burnout?

About the Facility's Philosophy of Care

The philosophy of the facility regarding care of residents with dementia is another important consideration. Answers to the following questions can be very telling about whether the facility is appropriate for your loved one:

- Are residents permitted to move about freely on the unit?
- Can they wander in and out of other resident's rooms? If not, how does the staff manage wandering behaviors?
- How are rummaging or hoarding behaviors handled?
- How are physically aggressive behaviors handled?
- How are verbal outbursts handled?
- How are sexual behaviors handled?
- What percentage of dementia residents are fed through a tube?
- What percentage of dementia residents need assistance with feeding or eating?
- Is there adequate staff to hand feed all residents in need of it?

Touring a Nursing Home
(Observations to Make During A Nursing Home Visit)

You might not be able to get the above information on a nursing home's website or by phone. Taking a tour of the facility is ultimately the best way to assess any prospective nursing home.

Touring a facility gives you the opportunity not only to ask pointed questions but also to observe the residents and staff and how they interact. On the other hand, it's difficult to tour a prospective nursing home with objectivity. I would urge you bring a friend or less involved family member who would be able not only to ask questions that might not occur to you but also to observe the surroundings more objectively than you or your family.

As you move through the facility, pay attention to the following:

Residents

- How do they look (happy, content, sad, agitated, etc.)?
- Do they interact with each other?
- Do you see residents up and about, walking either independently or with assistance, or residents in wheelchairs who are able to propel themselves?
- Do they appear clean and well groomed?
- Do the residents participate in the activities planned for them?

Staff-Patient Interaction

- Is there a lot of interaction or verbal communication between residents and staff?
- Does the staff behave as if they enjoy the residents they are caring for?
- How would you describe the interaction (friendly, familiar, authoritarian, etc.)?
- Do you sense a rapport between the staff and residents?

Facility

- What do hallways look like? For the most part, are they free of objects that could be hazardous to residents walking around?
- Are hallways and doorways wide enough for those residents who use walkers and wheelchairs to move about freely?
- Are the hallways equipped with handrails?
- Is the material on the floors nonskid?
- Are hallways, resident rooms, and common areas well lighted?
- Does the facility appear clean, cheerful, and safe?
- Are the hallways, rooms, bathrooms, and public spaces free from unpleasant odors?

- Is there a plan in place to adequately remove and dispose of all trash and soiled linen to decrease lingering odors?

Questions to Ask on Your Tour

Below are some suggestions for questions to ask during your tour that can help you choose, or reject, a nursing home. Many other questions might occur to you during the tour. Don't hesitate to ask them—the more information you can get the better.

- Which physician(s) will be caring for your loved one? Are they experienced in dealing with Alzheimer's patients?
- What can the family expect in regards to communication between the staff and family (updates, changes in status of family member, care conferences, etc.)?
- If there is an activities director on staff at the facility, what percentage of their week is dedicated to the dementia population? (Ask for examples of activities offered specifically to the dementia population.) If there isn't a dedicated activities director, who plans activities?
- When a new resident is admitted to the unit, what process is used to help them adjust to their new environment? Is there flexibility to meet the resident where they are behaviorally and cognitively, or is it expected they will have to adjust to an already established system? How does the nursing home staff achieve those goals with a new resident?

In addition, address specific problematic behaviors your loved one exhibits. For each behavior, ask if the nursing home considers it acceptable or not, and ask how they would manage the behavior or try to eliminate it.

As we began the search for a second nursing home, we asked an admissions coordinator if rummaging and wandering around the unit, including into other residents' rooms, was acceptable or not. It was a secure unit, exclusively for those residents with dementia. Dad and I were firmly but kindly told that neither behavior was acceptable and were promptly shown to the door. It was that experience and a few others like it that helped us identify what were nonnegotiable characteristics for the next nursing home we would choose for Mom. Even though we received the answers we were looking for from the admissions staff where Mom lives now, I was very concerned when Barb and I visited Mom for the first time and she was carrying around a blanket and pillow that didn't belong to her. Anxiously, I turned to Barb and expressed concern that Mom was going to find herself in trouble for this behavior. The nurse overheard me and I'll never forget what she said: "It's OK. Don't worry about it. Your mom's just been shopping. We'll return the pillow and blanket to their correct owner as soon as your mom's done holding them."

Conclusion

Sending your loved one to adult day care, bringing hired help (such as homecare or home healthcare) into your home, or moving your loved one to a care facility can be really painful decisions to make. All three highlight the progression of the disease in your loved one and the increased dependence on others for care. I suspect most, if not all, families and caregiving groups will struggle with these decisions at least a bit.

For the longest time, I viewed the decision to move Mom to a nursing home as the final decision we would have to make for her. In other words, Mom's move to the nursing home would be her final chapter. Not so. She has been living in a nursing home for several years and there are still decisions we face as her family caregivers, and there will be in the future as well. After observing Mom and the residents in her unit for the past five years, I've come to realize that the final chapter for each of them is unique, even though they all have dementia. That said, eating and feeding issues and whether or not to use CPR, to hospitalize, to consent to surgery, to treat infections with antibiotics, or to bring in hospice care are common end-stage Alzheimer's issues that many of us will have to face. In the next chapter, I will discuss those issues, as well as how to spend quality time with your loved one at the end of their life.

Resources

Finding an Adult Day Program

▶ **The Community Resource Finder**
The Community Resource Finder through the Alzheimer's Association allows you to access comprehensive listings of adult day programs, homecare, and home healthcare. You can also narrow results, looking at individual services an adult day program or homecare or home healthcare provider might offer.
www.communityresourcefinder.org/

▶ **The National Adult Day Services Association**
Following NADSA's step-by-step process will help you choose an adult day center for your loved one. In addition, their website can link you to pertinent research studies in the field of adult day care.
www.nadsa.org/

Finding Homecare or Home Healthcare

▶ **Medicare**
This is a good site to determine which home health agencies are Medicare program participants. An easy-to-read chart lets you quickly determine which services are offered for each home health agency listed. *Medicare-certified* indicates that the home health agency is approved by Medicare and meets certain federal health and safety requirements.
www.medicare.gov/homehealthcompare/search.html

▶ **The National Association for Home Care and Hospice**
The National Association for Home Care and Hospice has an agency locator that provides you with information on homecare agencies in an easy-to-understand format.
agencylocator.nahc.org/

▶ **Family Caregiver Alliance**
How to hire in-home help detailed in a fact- and tip-sheet format. Assessing homecare needs, finding the right homecare worker, and interviewing the applicant are a few of the topics addressed.
www.caregiver.org/fact-sheets

Finding a Residential Care Facility

▶ **The Alzheimer's Association** 1–800–272–3900
Detailed information about choosing a residential care facility, including what to look for, what to ask, types of care settings (retirement housing, assisted living, nursing homes, Alzheimer's specialty care units, continuing care retirement communities), and finding licensed facilities.
www.alz.org/care/alzheimers-dementia-care-housing.asp

▶ **The Community Resource Finder**
The Community Resource Finder allows you to access comprehensive listings of nursing homes. You can also narrow results, looking at individual services a nursing home might offer.
www.communityresourcefinder.org/

▶ **Medicare**
This is a good site to determine which residential care facilities are Medicare/Medicaid program participants and how they rate in state inspections (health inspections, staffing, and quality ratings).
www.medicare.gov/nursinghomecompare/search.html?

▶ **A Place for Mom**
Assistance in finding the right care facility for your loved one.
www.aplaceformom.com/

▶ **Peter Rabins Alzheimer's Family Support Center**
"The Nursing Home Decision—Memory and Alzheimer's Disease" (video)
www.youtube.com/watch?v=mv8qO-xR3bo&feature=youtu.be

Ten

The Final Chapter

I first noticed Mom struggling with her memory sixteen years ago. She was diagnosed with mild cognitive impairment two years later, and in 2006 she received the diagnosis of Alzheimer's disease. She has been living with the increasing effects of Alzheimer's disease for several years now and has been living in a nursing home for the past five years. Helpless to stop or even slow the relentless progression of this disease, my family and I have tried to soften the blow of what's to come. We strive both to provide loving care to Mom but also to ensure that she will continue receiving the best possible care so she is as comfortable as possible as her disease progresses.

Not surprisingly, my feelings about end-of-life care for those with Alzheimer's disease have been hugely influenced by the road I've walked with Mom. However, these are not easy issues to reconcile in your heart and mind. And because most of them are rooted in ethics, strong feelings and opinions might accompany the weighty decisions we all ultimately have to make. With that in mind, I'll make every effort to present the end-of-life issues in this chapter as objectively as I possibly can.

Advance Directives

Before getting into specifics, I want to readdress the issue of advance directives discussed in Chapter 3: Knowledge is Power. Has your loved one shared their desires through advanced directives? If so, are you prepared to honor them? In the absence of those directives, are you willing to look at the end-of-life decisions you might have to make and choose what you think your loved one would want even if that differs from your wishes? How do you want your loved one's last months, weeks, days and moments to be for them ... and for you?

Advance directives can include a living will and a durable power of attorney for healthcare. A living will is a written document that explains how a person wants to be treated if they are dying or permanently unconscious. A durable power of attorney appoints a proxy to make healthcare decisions for a person when they no longer can. The proxy must follow the wishes described in the living will or make decisions in the person's best interests if there is no living will. It's a good idea to have both in place while your loved one is still capable of making these decisions.[1]

Advance Directives can include directions on the following issues:

- CPR (cardiopulmonary resuscitation)
- DNR (do not resuscitate)
- DNH (do not hospitalize)
- Use of antibiotics
- Use of dialysis
- Use of a ventilator
- Artificial feeding
- Artificial hydration
- Treatment of pain
- Hospitalization

- Comfort or palliative care
- Hospice care

Advance Directives are usually in writing, though sometimes the living will portion is only verbally expressed. However, there can be differences from state to state. Some states will treat advance directives that are shared verbally as formal advance directives as long as they are witnessed properly.[2]

In either case, if your loved one has advance directives, you and your family are responsible for carrying out those wishes. If not, according to Viki Kind in her article "Avoiding the Pitfalls in CPR/DNR Decision Making," "as the decision maker, you are supposed to consider all that you know about your loved one, what he/she told you in the past, what their values are and what would be important to him/her. Using this information, you should do your best to make the decision you think your loved one would make."[3]

My mom is now in the advanced stages of Alzheimer's disease, so my family and I are confronting some difficult issues (and we will certainly be confronting others in the not-too-distant future). Among the issues you might face as your loved one's disease progresses are:

- What is the best way to nourish your loved one at this stage of their disease?
- Under what circumstances, if any, should your loved one undergo surgery or be hospitalized?
- Should infections be treated with antibiotics, or should only the symptoms be managed?
- When should you consider hospice care?

I will discuss these issues in more detail below. The information I include in this chapter is not meant to tell you what to do in any given circumstance. Rather, it's provided to assist you in making tough decisions, just as I believe it will be helpful in guiding my family when we have to make what will undoubtedly be difficult decisions.

Nutrition Issues

At one of the first care conferences we attended at Mom's nursing home, we were presented with some information regarding her weight or, more precisely, her weight loss. The dietician provided us with some numbers that had been steadily declining since her admission only a few months prior. The dietician explained that Mom was burning too many calories because of the large amount of time she walked and paced the halls of her unit. In addition, she rarely sat still long enough to eat an entire meal. And despite the recent addition of high-calorie supplements, Mom continued to lose weight.

The dietician offered us an option: to put a feeding (gastrostomy) tube into Mom's stomach. The tube, also known as a **PEG (percutaneous endoscopic gastrostomy) tube**, would help stabilize her weight by providing additional calories. Dad and I looked at each other and expressed our shared opinion to the dietician after a brief conversation that went something like this:

Amy: "She's an eighty-year-old woman with Alzheimer's living in a nursing home."

Dad: "No way."

Amy: "Mom wouldn't want that."

Dad: "Alzheimer's is a terminal disease after all."

In that moment, I didn't recall that Mom had a living will that spelled out her wishes in regards to being fed through a tube. But Dad did. He explained, "Dolores's living will states that she does not want to be kept alive by being fed through a tube or being hooked up to any other machines." Period.

Artificial Nutrition and Feeding Tubes

Eating and nutrition problems are common and expected, especially in late-stage Alzheimer's disease. While in Mom's case burning too many calories was the problem, many others with Alzheimer's disease have lower caloric needs due to a lower metabolic rate and decreased activity. But this nutrition problem is not exclusive to those with Alzheimer's disease. Eating and drinking less is a natural progression toward the end of life in many other terminal conditions.[4] Many times, however, the reaction from caregivers is to counteract the decrease in oral intake by inserting a feeding tube. In fact, about one in three nursing home residents with advanced dementia are tube fed, whether it's a tube going through one of the nostrils and down to the stomach (**nasogastric tube**) or a tube going directly into the stomach through the abdominal wall, like a PEG tube.[5] Considerable controversy surrounds this practice. Indeed, **artificial nutrition**, feeding tubes, and artificial hydration are among the most controversial issues in nursing-home care.

The cons of artificial nutrition include the possibility of:
- Discomfort from the tube
- Need for restraints to prevent tube removal
- Need for pharmacologic sedation
- Lack of enjoyment of oral intake of food
- Lack of contact with care providers during feeding
- Diminished quality of life

In addition, there are many potential side effects and complications from artificial feeding tubes. They include:
- Bleeding
- Perforation of the esophagus
- Infection
- Pain
- Aspiration into the lungs

- Skin irritation
- Edema
- Leaking around the tube
- Diarrhea
- Nausea and vomiting

With so many issues, why do feeding tubes end up being placed in so many patients with advanced dementia? I think caregivers want to feel they are doing all they can to care for their loved one's needs. Surely providing adequate nutrition is a cornerstone of caregiving. Plus, the reasons to support the use of a feeding tube can be compelling, especially if it comes from your loved one's healthcare providers. And there definitely are some pros to feeding tubes. For example, feeding tubes are helpful when the primary cause of the eating problem is likely to improve (i.e., recovering from stroke, brain injury, or surgery). Feeding tubes are also useful for patients with certain kinds of cancers, digestive disorders, and burns. In other words, they are beneficial for people who have problems swallowing but who are not in the last stage of an illness that can't be cured.

But when you consider a person in the advanced or final stage(s) of dementia, the research simply does not support the use of feeding tubes. According to the American Geriatrics Society, "feeding tubes are not recommended for older adults with advanced dementia. Careful hand feeding should be offered; efforts to enhance oral feeding by altering the environment and creating patient-centered approaches to feeding should be part of usual care for older adults with advanced dementia."[6]

Hand Feeding vs. Tube Feeding

As I mentioned above, eating and feeding problems are very common among people with Alzheimer's disease. Indeed, it's estimated that close to 90 percent of people with advanced dementia will develop these problems.[7] Problems with swallowing (**dysphagia**) are one of the reasons for these difficulties.

To understand swallowing problems, think back to when your loved one started having difficulties with activities such as driving and hygiene. If you're like me, that was the first time you examined the complexity of both of those tasks that are accomplished with ease by a person with a healthy brain. It wasn't until I started looking closely at the steps necessary to be a safe driver and to accomplish self-hygiene that I was able to grasp why Mom and others with Alzheimer's disease would increasingly struggle with these and other complex tasks, such as swallowing, as their dementia progressed.

We take it for granted, but swallowing is a complex behavior. Food and liquids are moved from the mouth to the stomach during swallowing. Multiple nerves and muscles are involved, both willfully and reflexively. An important function of swallowing is how the airway is protected from food and liquids entering into it. This aspect of swallowing is particularly concerning in the later stages of Alzheimer's disease. If this protective function no longer works, the person can choke. It's understandable, then, why adaptations would need to be made when your loved one has difficulty swallowing.

To minimize the risk of choking (and malnutrition), it's important to bring any eating difficulties to the attention of the staff (or their physician if your loved one is at home). A healthcare professional experienced in evaluating and treating eating and feeding difficulties might be recommended to address such issues as:

- Modifications to the texture, viscosity, and density of your loved one's food
- Adjustments to your loved one's posture and positioning while eating

- Fixing of dental problems, such as ill-fitting dentures
- Modifications to the environment during mealtime, such as eliminating external stimuli that could be distracting to your loved one

When we are specifically addressing the needs of a person in the late stages of Alzheimer's, what if we shifted our thinking away from tube feeding? Instead, we could take into account the individual feeding challenges our loved ones are experiencing, as well as the change in their nutritional needs near the end of life. At the same time, we could make mealtime as comfortable, comforting, and pleasurable for our loved ones as possible. This concept, known as **careful or comfort hand feeding**, is detailed in a 2010 article in the *Journal of the American Geriatrics Society*.[8] But careful hand feeding is not just a concept. I see it in action every time I visit Mom at the nursing home during mealtime. With this type of individualized feeding, your loved one's comfort during mealtime is the focus. As long as they don't show signs of coughing or choking, or other signs of distress, hand feeding should be encouraged. If medically safe, careful or comfort hand feeding can allow your loved one to continue to enjoy the pleasures of eating in the company of family, friends, and caring staff.

As I mentioned in Chapter 6: Safety First, Mom is not having problems with eating yet. She has always enjoyed eating, so this concept of comfort hand feeding is one that really resonates with me, especially given Mom's wishes, and we're fortunate to have her wishes detailed for us in her living will. She does not want to be fed through a tube. So some days she eats and drinks well and some days she doesn't. We have to be OK with that.

Hospitalization

Unfortunately, Mom's living will doesn't cover the issue of hospitalization. However, knowing how sensitive she now is to even the tiniest change in routine, I would be hard-pressed to agree to having her hospitalized unless it was the result of an injury, such as a laceration needing stitches or a broken bone.

People with advanced dementia are hospitalized more often than people of similar ages who are cognitively healthy or have milder dementia.[9] As a matter of fact, 25 percent of nursing home residents with advanced dementia will be hospitalized in the last six months of life.[10] However, many hospitalizations for nursing home residents with dementia could be avoided because nursing-home care has been shown to be as effective as hospital care for the treatment of many common conditions such as pneumonia.[11] In addition, the transfer of people with Alzheimer's disease from nursing homes to hospitals has been shown to result in distress, functional decline, and other problems including delirium, confusion, incontinence, and falls.[12] So the big question becomes, under what circumstances should our loved ones be hospitalized?

Pneumonia and Other Infections

The majority of hospitalizations among people with Alzheimer's disease are the result of **pneumonia** and other infections. Pneumonia is a breathing condition in which there is swelling or an infection of the lungs or large airways. The risk of pneumonia is increased in those with Alzheimer's disease as well as in those who are confined to bed or those who are tube fed.

The most common type of pneumonia among people with Alzheimer's disease is aspiration pneumonia, which occurs when food, saliva, liquids, or vomit is breathed into the lungs or the airways leading to the lungs. The incidence of aspiration pneumonia is increased in people with periodontal disease. Indeed, good oral care has shown to decrease the incidence of pneumonia and mortality from it.[13]

Viruses and bacteria can also cause pneumonia. While antibiotics can be effective in treating bacterial diseases, including pneumonia, they are useless for treating viral pneumonia and other viral diseases. Interestingly, hospitalization for pneumonia does not improve functional status or survival when compared to those treated on site. Indeed, immediate survival and mortality rates are similar if the infection is treated in a hospital vs. a long-term care facility, but the long-term outcomes are better for patients treated in a nursing home.[14]

Falls and Hip Fractures

Broken or fractured hips are another major cause of hospitalization (and death) among the elderly. Osteoporosis and falls are major risk factors for hip fractures. Falls are unfortunately quite common in with people with Alzheimer's disease and other forms of dementia. Indeed, their risk of falling is 20 to 30 percent greater than those without dementia, and they are almost three times more likely to fracture a hip.[15] Whether dementia is present or not, once a person has sustained a hip fracture, they have an increased risk of having a second one.[16] Sadly, most people who have had a hip fracture do not regain the level of independence they had before the injury. Approximately half will require a walker or some other device or assistance even after recovery.[17]

To that point, we made the decision to transition Mom to a wheelchair after she sustained a couple falls that, thankfully, didn't result in any broken bones but did require two trips to the emergency room for evaluation and treatment of scalp lacerations. Both the nursing home staff and my family decided to move Mom to the wheelchair before she did sustain a more serious injury.

Is there a way to guarantee that your loved one will not sustain a hip fracture? Not really. Even people who are bedridden or wheelchair-bound can sustain hip fractures. But there are ways to decrease the chances of your loved falling and fracturing a hip:

- Make sure your loved one's environment is safe (refer to the suggestions in Chapter 6: Safety First)
- Talk to your loved one's doctor about osteoporosis prevention and treatment options
- Although the reviews are mixed, explore the possibility of using a hip protector undergarment if your loved one is ambulatory
- Have a physical or occupational therapist assess whether a cane or walker is a safe addition for your loved one

Pain Management

How we experience pain or discomfort is a very personal thing. What I perceive as severe pain might be nothing more than a twinge to someone else. An estimated 45 to 85 percent of elderly people are in chronic pain. The difficulty for people with Alzheimer's disease or dementia is, while they can experience pain, how they convey that they are in pain can be severely altered.

If a person with Alzheimer's disease doesn't have the language skills to express their pain or discomfort, it can be manifested in other ways. However, even individuals with end-stage dementia might be able to respond *yes* or *no* to a question about the presence of pain. And facial expressions and behaviors are particularly useful in detecting pain in people with Alzheimer's disease or dementia.

Signs of Pain in People with Dementia[18]

Facial expressions
- Slight frown; sad frightened face
- Grimacing, wrinkled forehead
- Closed or tightened eyes
- Any distorted expression
- Rapid blinking

Verbalizations, vocalizations
- Sighing, moaning, groaning
- Grunting, chanting, calling out
- Noisy breathing
- Asking for help
- Verbally abusive

Body movements
- Rigid, tense body posture, guarding
- Fidgeting
- Increased pacing, rocking
- Restricted movement
- Gait or mobility changes
- Changes in interpersonal interactions
- Aggressive, combative, resisting care
- Decreased social interactions
- Socially inappropriate, disruptive
- Withdrawn

Changes in activity patterns or routines
- Refusing food, appetite change
- Increase in rest periods
- Sleep, rest pattern changes
- Sudden cessation of common routines
- Increased wandering

Mental status changes
- Crying or tears

- Increased confusion
- Irritability or distress

Recognition and treatment of pain presents a major challenge in this population. But just because your loved one doesn't have the words to express their pain or discomfort doesn't mean they're not hurting. Undiagnosed or under-diagnosed pain can lead to inadequate treatment or even no treatment at all. When pain isn't treated or is undertreated, it can cause a variety of behavioral problems, as evidenced by the long list above of signs of pain in people with dementia. Inadequately treated pain can also result in sleep disturbances. Given the number of people with dementia who have sleep disturbances, I can't help wondering if that number could be impacted with proper pain management. I'm not saying that pain is the only reason that those with dementia have sleep difficulties. But it could be one of the reasons. It's worth exploring.

If you think your loved one is in pain, talk to their physician about initiating a trial of pain medication. If the pain medication results in their behavior or sleep problems returning to normal, or their nonverbal signs of pain disappearing, it's likely that pain was a causative factor and pain medication might continue to be needed.

What to Ask the Doctor About End-of-Life Care

The Alzheimer's Association developed the following set of questions to ask your loved one's healthcare provider when deciding on the type of care you would choose or decline for them:[19]

- What is the treatment for?
- How will it help?
- What are the physical risks or discomforts?
- What are the emotional risks or discomforts?

- Does the treatment match what the person would have wanted?
- Are we doing all we can to uphold their dignity?
- Are we doing all we can to give the person the best quality of life?
- Is he or she in pain?
- What can be done to ease the pain?
- When is the best time to ask for hospice care?

Other End-of-Life Issues

I'll bet CPR (cardiopulmonary resuscitation), DNR (do not resuscitate) orders, and hospice care are issues that don't cross most people's minds until they're faced with making those tough decisions for their loved ones.

I know we'll be called upon to make decisions for Mom as she continues to decline. And the decisions we will make will most likely differ from what we would have chosen when she was early in the disease process. Although Mom didn't discuss every aspect of her future care with us, she was very clear that she doesn't want to be hooked up to any life-sustaining machines. So she won't be. Because she doesn't want to be resuscitated (by CPR) in the event that her heart stops beating or she stops breathing, she has a DNR order.

CPR & DNR

Cardiopulmonary Resuscitation (CPR) is an emergency intervention used when a person's heart, breathing, or both stop. Mouth-to-mouth breathing provides oxygen to the lungs and brain, and chest compressions simulate the pumping action of the heart thus causing blood to circulate throughout the body.[20]

Do Not Resuscitate (DNR) is a medical order not to initiate CPR should a patient's heart stop beating or their breathing stop. A DNR order is written by a physician based on the wishes of the patient or their family. However, a DNR order only applies to CPR. Other medical treatments (such as artificial feeding) or pain and medications are not covered in a DNR order.[21]

Some important things to keep in mind when making a decision about CPR:

- CPR is three times less likely to be successful in a person with dementia than in one who is cognitively intact[22]
- With CPR, there is a chance of broken ribs, a collapsed lung, and damage to the windpipe
- The longer CPR takes, the longer your loved one will be without oxygen, and the greater the risk of further brain damage

If you're still undecided about CPR, consider whether it will increase the likelihood that your loved one will survive their illness, even if they survive CPR. CPR has been shown to be ineffective in increasing long-term survival in frail, elderly patients like those typically suffering from dementia. Those who do survive (between 0 and 2 percent) are in worse condition than before their hearts stopped.[23] In fact, doing CPR on an elderly, debilitated Alzheimer's patient might do more harm than good. According to Doug Smucker, MD, a professor of family medicine at the University of Cincinnati Health Sciences Center: "The chance that [CPR] would even work for such a patient is extremely low. The chance that it would return the patient to his or her former quality of life is practically nil."[24]

Hospice and Palliative Care

Hospice care is end-of-life care provided by an interdisciplinary team of healthcare professionals and volunteers to patients who have six months or less to live. Patients are given medical, psychological, and spiritual support with the goal of helping them have peace, comfort, and dignity during their final months. Hospice caregivers try to control pain and other symptoms so a person can remain as alert and comfortable as possible. Hospice programs also provide services to support a patient's family.

Focused on caring, not curing, hospice neither hastens nor postpones death. Hospice is a concept of care rather than a specific place, and it can take place at home or in a hospice center, skilled nursing facility, or hospital.

Palliative care is treatment of the discomfort, symptoms, and stress of serious illness. The goal of palliative care is to make patients feel comfortable, alleviate their suffering, and improve their quality of life. Palliative care is an integral and essential component of hospice care.

Palliative care provides relief from distressing problems such as:[25]

- Pain
- Shortness of breath
- Fatigue
- Constipation
- Nausea
- Loss of appetite
- Problems with sleep
- Drug and other treatment side effects

Both hospice and palliative care are provided by interdisciplinary teams of doctors, nurses, pharmacists, nutritionists, social workers, and volunteers. While hospice care always includes palliative care, the reverse is not true. Palliative care can be provided to patients of any age at any stage of their illness, whether the illness is curable or not. Or as PalliativeDoctors. org puts it, "hospice care is always palliative, but not all palliative care is hospice care."[26]

Who Qualifies for Hospice Care?

Hospice care, unlike palliative care, is limited to patients at the end of their lives. Patients must be considered terminally ill and have a life expectancy of six months or less to qualify for admission. To qualify for the Medicare benefit for hospice care or for coverage by many other insurance plans, patients must also be assessed by the hospice medical director in consultation with the patient's attending physician (if the individual has one) for appropriateness of admission to hospice.

Because it's often difficult to determine if a person has six months or less to live, the National Hospice and Palliative Care Organization (NHPCO) has published the following guidelines for admitting dementia patients.[27]

The patient should:
- Be unable to ambulate without assistance
- Be unable to dress without assistance
- Be unable to bathe without assistance
- Have intermittent or constant urinary or fecal incontinence
- Have difficulty speaking or being understood.
- During the previous 12 months, the patient should have had one of the following:
  - Aspiration pneumonia
  - A kidney infection or other upper urinary tract infection
  - Septicemia (blood infection)
  - Bed sores
  - Recurrent fevers after antibiotic therapy
- Insufficient calorie and fluid intake with a 10% weight loss in the previous 6 months.

While there are other guidelines used to establish criteria for admittance of Alzheimer's patients into hospice, at present Medicare uses the above NHPCO guidelines to evaluate hospice eligibility for Alzheimer's patients. (Other terminal conditions have different eligibility guidelines).

Even with these criteria, it's difficult to predict when a person with Alzheimer's disease will have six months or less to live. Indeed, there's considerable disagreement in published studies about what is considered a reliable predictor of six-month mortality as it relates to hospice eligibility.

Why is it so difficult to predict six-month mortality in Alzheimer's disease? For one, Alzheimer's disease can last many years. According to the Alzheimer's Association, on average, those with Alzheimer's disease live eight years after their symptoms become noticeable to others, but survival can range from four to twenty years. And second, age and other health conditions impact mortality for those with Alzheimer's disease. More than half of older adults have three or more chronic diseases such as heart disease, diabetes, and cancer with distinctive cumulative negative effects.[28]

Because it's so difficult to predict six-month mortality, doctors are often hesitant to refer patients to hospice. So what can we do as caregivers? For one thing, we need to keep the lines of communication open between ourselves and our loved one's physician(s) and healthcare providers regarding hospice and other relevant end-of-life issues even before we think it's needed.

We also need to:

- Be knowledgeable about what hospice can offer our loved ones and ourselves
- Become comfortable talking about hospice within our families and caregiving groups
- Continue acting as our loved one's advocate for the best possible care

Finally, even if our loved ones are not yet deemed eligible for hospice based on existing guidelines, we have every right to insist on a philosophy of care that might be more closely aligned to what we want for our loved ones in the advanced stages of Alzheimer's disease (at least until they are eligible for hospice care).

Does Hospice Care Make a Difference?

Research indicates that hospice care can make a positive difference for both patients and their families. A small study entitled "Association between Hospice Care and Psychological Outcomes in Alzheimer's Spousal Caregivers" confirms what you might expect: hospice does help alleviate some of the stress experienced during the end of a patient's life, and the study even suggests that there is a relationship between hospice care and caregiver psychological well-being.[29] In addition, another study entitled, "Does Hospice Improve Quality of Care for Persons Dying from Dementia?" bereaved family members were asked to evaluate the quality of care their loved ones received at the end of their lives up until death. Almost half of the respondents had loved ones who received hospice services. Those who received hospice services perceived a higher quality of care and quality of dying for their loved ones compared with the families of patients without hospice care. More specifically, hospice services were associated with fewer unmet needs, fewer reported concerns about the quality of care, and higher family ratings of the quality of care than with standard care. Pain management and breathing difficulties, in particular, were two areas that received higher satisfaction scores by families with hospice services than those without.[30]

In addition, compared with other bereaved families, those family members with hospice services reported being better informed about what to expect while their loved ones were dying, having more frequent emotional support before their loved one's death, and having better communication between staff and family. Not surprisingly, bereaved family members who received hospice services "at the right time" had lower problem scores than those who did not receive hospice services. What I found interesting, though, was that respondents who indicated that hospice services were implemented "too late" had higher problem scores than if hospice care was never used.[31] That's certainly something to consider when deciding on hospice care for your loved one.

My mom's disease is a progressive one and I know that hospice care is a choice my family and I might have to make for her. I've observed hospice care in action many times during the years Mom has been living in the nursing home. In addition, I'm honored to be a volunteer at a local hospice in Cincinnati. I'm humbled time and time again by the tender care provided to patients and their families. With that in mind, I need to amend my previous comment. Hospice care is a choice my family and I will want to make for Mom.

Spending Time Together

Mom has slowed down. She walks only when there is someone available to help her, but even with help, she is much less steady on her feet than before. Nonetheless, she uses a wheelchair to get around now, cruising independently through the halls. Mom has an irrepressible need to move, and the safety of being in her wheelchair allows her to satisfy that need.

Mom is also dependent on others for many things, whether it's dressing, bathing, toileting, or eating. And her language skills continue to decline, with made-up words taking the place of real ones with ever-increasing frequency.

But, in spite of it all and relatively speaking, Mom still has quality to her life. She continues to recognize her family as people she loves, whether she's aware of our relationship to her or not. Yes, she has bad days when there is nothing anyone can do to improve her mood or relieve her anxiety and irritability. Thankfully, those days are still outnumbered by days when she is contented (some of the time) and funny and social (more often than not). So far.

However, I'm keenly aware that Mom's disease is a progressive one. And because of that, I'm thankful for her good days and the time we can spend together.

Depending on your loved one's level of functioning, there are a number of activities you can do together and both enjoy. Make a list of your loved one's favorite activities and then explore ways you could incorporate them into their life now. Below are some activities you might consider:

- Taking a walk or car ride
- Singing familiar songs
- Listening to music or nature sounds
- Reading familiar stories or scripture
- Reciting familiar prayers
- Looking at old photo albums and family pictures
- Watching a favorite TV program or listening to a favorite radio program
- Sharing a favorite food (such as ice cream)
- Sitting quietly with each other and holding hands
- Offering caring touch (scratching back, stroking hair, or massaging hands)

Lastly, slow down and just be with each other. No matter what abilities and functions remain or cease to remain, being with your loved one during this time can be deeply meaningful for you both. Until someone can give irrefutable evidence that proves a person even in the most advanced stage of Alzheimer's disease has absolutely no awareness of anything, I hold tight to my belief that our presence *does* have meaning on some level to our loved ones.

Conclusion

I've had the hardest time trying to find a way to end this book gracefully. I believe part of my difficulty is that Mom is still alive. She's been living in a nursing home for several years and, as I mentioned above, has taken a couple falls that have resulted in two trips to the emergency room. Thankfully, those falls only resulted in some cuts and bruises. As a result, though, she spends her waking hours in a wheelchair if there is no one available to assist her with walking. While her language skills have declined tremendously, she vocalizes with heartfelt determination, attempting to stay connected to people. And her physical health remains strong.

Outside the walls of Mom's memory-care unit, life goes on for my family and me. We've learned to live with the grief that inescapably accompanies those who love someone with Alzheimer's disease. It ebbs and flows in each of us. However, from time to time and without warning, the sadness envelops me and I acknowledge that losing my mom this way is literally heartbreaking.

But I know I'm not alone feeling this way and neither are you. And while there is comfort in the connectedness you and I share being Alzheimer's disease caregivers, that doesn't make up for our need to be supported regularly in our day-to-day lives. My sincerest hope is that you and your loved one have a group of supporters, whether it be two or twenty, to lean on throughout this journey.

Resources

Making End-of-Life Decisions

▶ **The Alzheimer's Association** 1–800–272–3900
"End-of-Life Decisions: Honoring the Wishes of a
Person with Alzheimer's Disease"
www.alz.org/care/alzheimers-late-end-stage-
caregiving.asp

▶ **Family Caregiver Alliance Fact Sheets**
- "Advanced Illness: Holding On and Letting Go"
- "End-of-Life Decision Making"
- "Advanced Illness: Feeding Tubes and Ventilators"
- "Advanced Illness: CPR and DNR"
- "When Caregiving Ends"

www.caregiver.org/fact-sheets

▶ **Books**
*Hard Choices for Loving People: CPR, Feeding Tubes,
Palliative Care, Comfort Measures, and the Patient with
a Serious Illness*, 6th ed. by Hank Dunn (Quality of Life
Publishing, 2016)

My dad and I were given this book by one of the social
workers at Mom's nursing home. We were discussing
feeding tubes in a care conference and the social
worker thought this book would be helpful in guiding
us as we faced end-of-life issues with Mom. It has
been.

▶ **Videos**
"Witnessing Death: A Grandson's Reflections on
Alzheimer's" by David Rosenthal (available on
Amazon Video or as a DVD)

Finding Hospice and Palliative Care Organizations

▶ **The Community Resource Finder**
www.communityresourcefinder.org/

▶ **The National Hospice and**
Palliative Care Organization
www.nhpco.org/resources

▶ **Hospice Foundation of America**
hospicefoundation.org/Hospice-Directory

Glossary

Advance directives: "[D]ocuments that communicate the health care wishes of a person. These decisions are then carried out after the person no longer can make decisions. In most cases, these documents must be prepared while the person is legally able to execute them." A living will or durable power of attorney are examples of documents that might include the final health care wishes of your loved one.[1]

Alzheimer's disease: An incurable disease in which nerve cells in the brain deteriorate and brain matter becomes smaller. As a result, thinking, behavior, and memory are impaired.

Amyloid: A protein found in the brains of people with Alzheimer's disease. It builds up into *plaque* or *tangles*.

Artificial nutrition: Nutrition provided by nasal feeding tube or a tube inserted into the wall of the stomach (called a PEG tube).

Careful or comfort hand feeding: Hand feeding a person with swallowing difficulties in order to allow them the pleasure of eating rather than simply meeting caloric needs.

CAT (computerized axial tomography) scan: a type of x-ray that produces multiple images of the inside of the body.

Cerebral cortex: "the part of the brain most directly responsible for consciousness, with essential roles in perception, memory, thought, mental ability, and intellect, [as well as being] responsible for initiating voluntary activity."[2]

Clinical trial: A research study involving humans that rigorously tests safety, side effects, and how well a medication or behavioral treatment works.

Cognitive abilities: Perception, reasoning, judgment, acts of creativity, comprehension, memory, and learning are examples.

CPR (cardiopulmonary resuscitation): Administering breaths and chest compressions to someone who has stopped breathing and whose heart has stopped beating in the hopes of saving their life.

Cueing: The practice of providing clues, hints or suggestions, or prompts to assist a person with memory loss.

Delusions: False ideas that, in spite of proof to the contrary, are strongly believed.

Dementia: Not a disease unto itself, but a term that describes a group of symptoms such as changes in mood, behavior, and personality, as well as impaired thinking, memory, and reasoning that interfere with a person's day-to-day functioning.

DNH (do not hospitalize): Advance directive instructing healthcare providers not to hospitalize a person under certain conditions.

DNR (do not resuscitate): Advance directive instructing healthcare providers not to administer CPR in the event that a person's heart has stopped beating or they are not breathing.

Drug Trials:

> **Phase I** – Researchers test a new drug or treatment in a small group of people (twenty to eighty) for the first time to evaluate its safety, determine a safe dosage range, and identify side effects.

> **Phase II** – The drug or treatment is given to a larger group of people (several hundred) to see if it is effective and to further evaluate its safety.

> **Phase III** – The drug or treatment is given to large groups of people (several hundred to several thousand) to confirm its effectiveness, monitor side effects, compare it to commonly used treatments, and collect information that will allow the drug or treatment to be used safely.

Dysphagia: Problems with swallowing.

Early-onset Alzheimer's disease: Diagnosed before the age of sixty-five. A small percentage of those diagnosed with early-onset Alzheimer's disease have a rare gene that directly causes Alzheimer's, known as *familial Alzheimer's disease*.

Geriatric care manager: Typically healthcare professionals with nursing, social work, gerontology, or mental health backgrounds. They perform an assessment and create a care plan for your family moving forward, taking into account your family's specific challenges.

Hallucinations: Sights, sounds, sensations, tastes, or smells that do not really exist but that are experienced by the dementia patient as real.

Hoarding: The act of collecting items and hiding or storing them away.

Home health aides: Healthcare providers (usually trained and state certified) capable of helping with bathing, dressing, transferring, toileting, and feeding people with dementia.

Hospice care: End-of-life care provided by an interdisciplinary team of healthcare professionals and volunteers to patients who have six months or less to live. Patients are given medical, psychological, and spiritual support with the goal of helping them have peace, comfort, and dignity during their final months. Hospice caregivers try to control pain and other symptoms so a person can remain as alert and comfortable as possible. Hospice programs also provide services to support a patient's family.

Licensed health professionals: Healthcare providers trained and licensed to provide more advanced medical care including giving injections.

Mild cognitive impairment: More severe than the expected cognitive decline of normal aging, but less severe than dementia. It might be noticeable to family and close friends, but is usually not severe enough to interfere with daily activities.

Mini-mental state examination: Short-term memory, long-term memory, orientation, writing, and language are cognitive skills that are measured in this mental status exam.

MRI (magnetic resonance imaging): Noninvasive imaging using a magnetic field and radio frequency pulses to reveal changes in soft tissues, bones, and internal organs.

Nasogastric tube: A tube inserted through one of the nostrils and down into the stomach. Used to provide artificial nutrition.

Neurofibrillary tangles: Inside nerve cells, accumulated fragments of twisted protein (tau protein) accumulate.

Neuropsychological testing: Language, visual-perceptual skills, memory, attention, problem solving, and reasoning are tested to evaluate brain function and a person's capabilities.

Palliative care: Treatment of the discomfort, symptoms, and stress of serious illness. The goal of palliative care is to make patients feel comfortable, alleviate their suffering, and improve their quality of life. Palliative care is an integral and essential component of hospice care.

PEG (percutaneous endoscopic gastronomy) tube: A tube inserted directly into the stomach through the abdominal wall. Used to provide artificial nutrition.

PET (positron emission tomography) scan: a type of scan that looks for changes in the soft tissues using a radioactive dye injected through a vein in the arm.

Pneumonia: A breathing condition in which there is swelling or an infection of the lungs or large airways.

Rummaging: Searching through places where things are stored (for example, cabinets, drawers, closets, or the refrigerator).

Senile plaques: protein fragments that build up between nerve cells (also known as beta-amyloid).

Skilled healthcare professionals: Healthcare providers including nurses, physical therapists, occupational therapists, and speech therapists. Depending on their training, they might be able to perform many health-related tasks, such as changing bandages and dressings and assisting with medication administration. They might also offer various types of therapy such as physical, occupational, and speech.

Sundowning/sundown syndrome: Beginning in the late afternoon and into the night, many people with Alzheimer's disease experience *sundowning* symptoms, which include agitation, pacing, irritability, and disorientation.

Notes

Chapter One: Alzheimer's Disease: The Basics

1. Alzheimer's Disease International, "Alois Alzheimer," accessed March 5, 2017, alz.co.uk/alois-alzheimer.

2. Alzheimer's Disease International, "Alois Alzheimer."

3. O. Buda, et al., "Georges Marinesco and the Early Research in Neuropathology," *Neurology* 72, no. 1 (January 6, 2009): 88, doi:10.1212/01.wnl.0000338626.93425.74.

4. Alzheimer's Disease International, "Alois Alzheimer."

5. Alzheimer's Disease International, "Alois Alzheimer."

6. David Shenk, "The Memory Hole," *The New York Times* online, November 3, 2006, accessed May 2, 2017, http://www.nytimes.com/2006/11/03/opinion/03shenk.html.

7. J. M. S. Pearce, "Alzheimer's Disease," *Journal of Neurology, Neurosurgery & Psychiatry* 68, no. 3 (March 1, 2000): 348, doi:10.1136/jnnp.68.3.348.

8. BrightFocus Foundation, "Alzheimer's Disease Research and Education," accessed March 5, 2017, http://www.brightfocus.org/alzheimers.

9. Alzheimer's Association: Research Center, "Alzheimer's & Brain Research Milestones," accessed March 5, 2017, http://alz.org/research/science/major_milestones_in_alzheimers.asp.

10. Alzheimer's Association: Research Center, "Alzheimer's & Brain Research Milestones."

11. Alzheimer's Association: Research Center, "Alzheimer's & Brain Research Milestones."

12. National Institute on Aging, "NIA Timeline," accessed February 5, 2017, https://www.nia.nih.gov/about/nia-timeline.

13. National Institute on Aging, "NIA Timeline."

14. Alzheimer's Association: Research Center, "Alzheimer's & Brain Research Milestones."

15. Marlene Cimons, "FDA Approves First Alzheimer's Disease Treatment Medication," *The Tech* 113, no. 40 (September 10, 1993), accessed February 2, 2017, http://tech.mit.edu/V113/N40/fda.40w.html.

16. Alzheimer's Association: Research Center, "Alzheimer's & Brain Research Milestones."

17. US Department of Health and Human Services, "Estimates of Funding for Various Research, Condition, and Disease Categories (RCDC)," NIH Categorical Spending: NIH Research Portfolio Online Reporting Tools, published February 10, 2016, accessed March 5, 2017, https://report.nih.gov/categorical_spending.aspx.

18. Cleveland Clinic, "Alzheimer's Disease Glossary of Terms," accessed March 5, 2017, http://my.clevelandclinic.org/health/articles/alzheimers-disease-glossary-of-terms.

19. Cleveland Clinic, "Alzheimer's Disease Glossary of Terms."

20. ClinicalTrials.gov, "Learn About Clinical Studies," accessed May 9, 2017, https://clinicaltrials.gov/ct2/about-studies/learn#ClinicalTrials.

21. Cleveland Clinic, "Alzheimer's Disease Glossary of Terms."

22. Cleveland Clinic, "Alzheimer's Disease Glossary of Terms."

23. Cleveland Clinic, "Alzheimer's Disease Glossary of Terms."

24. National Institutes of Health, "The Basics," accessed May 9, 2017, https://www.nih.gov/health-information/nih-clinical-research-trials-you/basics.

25. Alzheimer's Association, "Younger-Onset Alzheimer's & Dementia," Accessed March 5, 2017. https://www.alz.org/alzheimers_disease_early_onset.asp.

26. Cleveland Clinic, "Alzheimer's Disease Glossary of Terms."

27. Mayo Clinic, "Mild Cognitive Impairment," accessed March 5, 2017, http://www.mayoclinic.org/diseases-conditions/mild-cognitive-impairment/home/ovc-20206082.

28. Cleveland Clinic, "Alzheimer's Disease Glossary of Terms."

29. Cleveland Clinic, "Alzheimer's Disease Glossary of Terms."

30. Cleveland Clinic, "Alzheimer's Disease Glossary of Terms."

31. Alzheimer's Association, "What Is Alzheimer's?" accessed March 5, 2017, alz.org/alzheimers_disease_what_is_alzheimers.asp#tangles.

32. National Institute on Aging, "Rummaging and Hiding Things: Alzheimer's Caregiving Tips," accessed March 5, 2017, https://www.nia.nih.gov/alzheimers/publication/rummaging-and-hiding-things.

33. Alzheimer's Association: New York Chapter, "The Hard End of the Day: Shedding New Light on Sundowning," *Advancing Care Newsletter* (January/February 2012), accessed March 5, 2017, http://www.alznyc.org/nyc/advancingcare/janfeb2012.asp.

Chapter 2: Getting a Diagnosis

1. Alzheimer's Association, "Alzheimer's and Dementia Testing for Earlier Diagnosis," accessed March 5, 2017, http://www.alz.org/research/science/earlier_alzheimers_diagnosis.asp.

2. Alzheimer's Association, "10 Early Signs and Symptoms of Alzheimer's," accessed March 5, 2017, http://www.alz.org/alzheimers_disease_10_signs_of_alzheimers.asp. Used with permission from the Alzheimer's Association.

Chapter 3: Knowledge Is Power

1. Alzheimer's Disease Education & Referral (ADEAR) Center, "Legal and Financial Planning for People with Alzheimer's Disease: Fact Sheet," PDF, updated August 2010, https://www.nia.nih.gov/alzheimers/topics/legal-and-financial-planning.

2. P. Triplett, et al, "Content of Advance Directives for Individuals with Advanced Dementia," Journal of Aging and Health 20, no. 5 (August 2008): table 3, doi:10.1177/0898264308317822.

3. The Alzheimer's Association, "Strategic Plan," accessed March 6, 2017, http://www.alz.org/about_us_strategic_plan.asp.

Chapter 4: Communication Strategies

1. National Institute on Aging, "Caring for a Person with Alzheimer's Disease: Your Easy-to-Use Guide from the National Institute on Aging," PDF, accessed March 5, 2017, https://www.nia.nih.gov/sites/.../caring_for_a_person_with_alzheimers_disease_0.pdf.

Chapter 5: Help with Hygiene

1. Takeyoshi Yoneyama, DDS, PhD, et al, "Oral Care Reduces Pneumonia in Older Patients in Nursing Homes," Journal of the American Geriatrics Society 50, no. 3 (April 2002): 432, accessed March 6, 2017, https://www.researchgate.net/publication/11423562_Oral_care_reduces_pneumonia_in_older_patients_in_nursing_homes.

Chapter 6: Help with Hygiene

1. Alzheimer's Association, "Driving," PDF, accessed March 5, 2017, https://www.alz.org/documents/greaterillinois/driving.pdf.

Chapter 7: Coping with Disturbing Behaviors and Emotions

1. National Institute on Aging, "Caring for a Person with Alzheimer's Disease."

Chapter 8: Caregiver Survival

1. Alzheimer's Association, "2017 Alzheimer's Disease Facts and Figures: Quick Facts," accessed March 17, 2017, http://www.alz.org/facts/.

2.   National Institute on Aging, "Caregiver Guide: Tips for
     Caregivers of People with Alzheimer's Disease," PDF, 15,
     accessed March 5, 2017, https://www.bu.edu/alzresearch/
     files/pdf/NIAcaregiverguide03-073.pdf.

Chapter 9: Getting the Best Care for Your Loved One

1.   Alzheimer's Association, "Adult Day Centers," accessed
     March 20, 2017, https://www.alz.org/care/alzheimers-de-
     mentia-adult-day-centers.asp. Used with permission from
     the Alzheimer's Association.

2.   Adapted with permission from the Alzheimer's Associa-
     tion, "Choosing Care Providers," accessed March 20,
     2017, www.alz.org/care/alzheimers-dementia-screening-
     providers.asp.

3.   Alzheimer's Association, "Choosing Care Providers."
     Used with permission from the Alzheimer's Association.

4.   Adapted with permission from Alzheimer's Association,
     "Residential Care," accessed March 21, 2017, http://www.
     alz.org/care/alzheimers-dementia-residential-facilities.
     asp#choosing.

Chapter 10: The Final Chapter

1.   National Institute on Aging, "Advance Care Planning,"
     accessed March 21, 2017, https://www.nia.nih.gov/health/
     publication/advance-care-planning#wishes.

2.   Charles P. Sabatino, "10 Legal Myths About Advance
     Medical Directives," accessed March 13, 2017, http://www.
     pluk.org/ITVdocs/PFT_12-03-07_materials.pdf.

3.   Accessed March, 21, 2017, http://kindethics.
     com/2010/09/10-pitfalls-to-avoid-in-dnr-decision-mak-
     ing/.

4. Crossroads Hospice and Palliative Care, "Hospice Care Guidance: Nutrition at the End of Life," accessed April 26, 2017, https://www.crossroadshospice.com/caregiver-guidance/nutrition-hydration.

5. Howard Brody, MD, PhD, et al., "Artificial Nutrition and Hydration: The Evolution of Ethics, Evidence, and Policy," *Journal of General Internal Medicine* 26, no. 9 (September 2011): 1053, doi:10.1007/s11606-011-1659-z.

6. American Geriatrics Society (AGS), "Feeding Tubes in Advanced Dementia Position Statement," accessed March 6, 2017, http://www.americangeriatrics.org/files/documents/feeding.tubes.advanced.dementia.pdf.

7. Laura C. Hanson, et al., "Oral Feeding Options for Patients with Dementia: A Systematic Review." Journal of the American Geriatrics Society 59, no. 3 (March 2011): 463, accessed March 6, 2017, https://www.ncbi.nlm.nih.gov/pmc/articles/PMC3164780/.

8. Erik J. Palecek, MSIV, et al., "Comfort Feeding Only: A Proposal to Bring Clarity to Decision-Making Regarding Difficulty with Eating for Persons with Advanced Dementia," *Journal of the American Geriatrics Society* 58, no. 3 (March 2010): 580–84, doi:10.1111/j.1532-5415.2010.02740.x.

9. Ladislav Volicer, MD, PhD, "End-of-Life Care for People with Dementia in Residential Care Settings," PDF from the Alzheimer's Association, accessed March 6, 2017, https://www.alz.org/documents/national/endoflifelitreview.pdf.

10. Jane L. Givens, MD, et al., "Hospital Transfers Among Nursing Home Residents with Advanced Dementia," *Journal of the American Geriatrics Society* 60, no. 5 (May 2012): 905, doi:10.1111/j.1532-5415.2012.03919.x.

11. Givens, et al., "Hospital Transfers," 905.

12. Volicer, "End-of-Life Care," 3.

13. Takeyoshi Yoneyama, DDS, PhD, et al., "Oral Care Reduces Pneumonia in Older Patients," 432.

14. Volicer, "End-of-Life Care," 3.

15. Isaura B. Menzies, et al., "Prevention and Clinical Management of Hip Fractures in Patients with Dementia," *Geriatric Orthopedic Surgery & Rehabilitation* 1, no. 2 (November 2010): 63 and 65, doi:10.1177/2151458510389465.

16. Menzies, "Prevention and Clinical Management," 67.

17. Cleveland Clinic, "Hip Fracture," accessed March 6, 2017, http://my.clevelandclinic.org/health/articles/hip-fracture.

18. American Geriatrics Society Panel on Persistent Pain in Older Persons (2002), "The Management of Persistent Pain in Older Persons," *Journal of the American Geriatrics Society* 50, no. 6 (June 2002 supplement): 211. Used with permission from the American Geriatrics Society.

19. Alzheimer's Association, "End-of-Life Decisions: Honoring the Wishes of a Person with Alzheimer's Disease," PDF, accessed March 6, 2017, http://www.alz.org/national/documents/brochure_endoflifedecisions.pdf. Used with permission from the Alzheimer's Association.

20. Hank Dunn, *Hard Choices for Loving People: CPR, Feeding Tubes, Palliative Care, Comfort Measures, and the Patient with a Serious Illness,* 5th ed. (Lansdowne, VA: A & A Publishers, 2009), 13.

21. Medline Plus, "Do-Not-Resuscitate Order," accessed March 6, 2017, https://medlineplus.gov/ency/patientinstructions/000473.htm.

22. Volicer, "End-of-Life Care," 2.

23. Dunn, *Hard Choices,* 13 and 15.

24. Marie Marley, "Make Alzheimer's End-of-Life Healthcare Decisions Long Before You Need Them," *Huffpost: The Blog,* May 22, 2012, http://www.huffingtonpost.com/marie-marley/alzheimers_b_1436702.html.

25. The National Institute of Nursing Research, "Palliative Care: The Relief You Need When You're Experiencing the Symptoms of Serious Illness," accessed March 6, 2017, https://www.ninr.nih.gov/sites/default/files/Palliative-Care-Relief-When-Experiencing-Symptoms-Serious-Illness-508.pdf.

26. "Frequently Asked Questions about Hospice and Palliative Care," accessed March 22, 2017, http://palliativedoctors.org/faq.

27. Ronald S. Schonwetter, MD, et al., "Predictors of Six-Month Survival Among Patients with Dementia: An Evaluation of Hospice Medicare Guidelines," *American Journal of Hospice and Palliative Medicine* 20, no. 2 (March–April 2003): 107, doi:10.1177/104990910302000208.

28. American Geriatrics Society Expert Panel on the Care of Older Adults with Multimorbidity, "Patient-Centered Care for Older Adults."

29. S. Irwin, et al., "Association Between Hospice Care and Psychological Outcomes in Alzheimer's Spousal Caregivers," *Journal of Palliative Medicine* 16, no. 11 (November 2013): 1453, doi:10.1089/jpm.2013.0130.

30. Joan M. Teno, MD, MS, et al., "Does Hospice Improve Quality of Care for Persons Dying from Dementia?" NIH Public Access Author Manuscript, 10, accessed May 9, 2017, https://www.ncbi.nlm.nih.gov/pmc/articles/PMC3724341/pdf/nihms480027.pdf.

31. Teno, et al., "Does Hospice Care Improve Quality," 4.

Glossary

1. National Institute on Aging, "Advance Care Planning."

2. Laurence Urdan, *The Bantam Medical Dictionary,* 3rd rev. ed. (New York: Bantam, 2000), s.v. "cerebral cortex."

References

Alzheimer's Association. "Adult Day Centers." Accessed March 20, 2017. https://www.alz.org/care/alzheimers-dementia-adult-day-centers.asp.

———. "Alzheimer's and Dementia Testing for Earlier Diagnosis." Accessed March 5, 2017. http://www.alz.org/research/science/earlier_alzheimers_diagnosis.asp.

———. "Choosing Care Providers." Accessed March 20, 2017. https://www.alz.org/care/alzheimers-dementia-screening-providers.asp.

———. "Driving." PDF. Accessed March 5, 2017. https://www.alz.org/documents/greaterillinois/driving.pdf.

———. "End-of-Life Decisions: Honoring the Wishes of a Person with Alzheimer's Disease." Accessed March 6, 2017. http://www.alz.org/national/documents/brochure_endoflifedecisions.pdf.

———. "Residential Care." Accessed March 21, 2017. http://www.alz.org/care/alzheimers-dementia-residential-facilities.asp#choosing.

———. "Strategic Plan." Accessed March 6, 2017. http://www.alz.org/about_us_strategic_plan.asp.

————. "10 Early Signs and Symptoms of Alzheimer's." Accessed March 5, 2017. http://www.alz.org/alzheimers_ disease_10_signs_of_alzheimers.asp.

————. "2017 Alzheimer's Disease Facts and Figures: Quick Facts." Accessed March 17, 2017. http://www.alz.org/facts/.

————. "What Is Alzheimer's?" Accessed March 5, 2017. alz. org/alzheimers_disease_what_is_alzheimers.asp#tangles.

————. "Younger-Onset Alzheimer's & Dementia." Accessed March 5, 2017. https://www.alz.org/alzheimers_disease_ early_onset.asp.

Alzheimer's Association: New York Chapter. "The Hard End of the Day: Shedding New Light on Sundowning." *Advancing Care Newsletter* (January/February 2012). Accessed March 5, 2017. http://www.alznyc.org/nyc/ advancingcare/janfeb2012.asp.

Alzheimer's Association: Research Center. "Alzheimer's & Brain Research Milestones." Accessed March 5, 2017. http://alz.org/research/science/major_milestones_in_ alzheimers.asp.

Alzheimer's Disease Education & Referral (ADEAR) Center. "Legal and Financial Planning for People with Alzheimer's Disease: Fact Sheet." PDF. Updated August 2010. https://www.nia.nih.gov/alzheimers/topics/legal- and-financial-planning.

Alzheimer's Disease International. "Alois Alzheimer." Accessed March 5, 2017. https://www.alz.co.uk/alois- alzheimer.

American Geriatrics Society (AGS). "Feeding Tubes in Advanced Dementia Position Statement." Accessed March 6, 2017. http://www.americangeriatrics.org/files/documents/feeding.tubes.advanced.dementia.pdf.

American Geriatrics Society Panel on Persistent Pain in Older Persons (2002). "The Management of Persistent Pain in Older Persons." *Journal of the American Geriatrics Society* 50, no. 6 (June 2002 supplement): 5205–24.

American Geriatrics Society Expert Panel on the Care of Older Adults with Multimorbidity. "Patient-Centered Care for Older Adults with Multiple Chronic Conditions: A Stepwise Approach from the American Geriatrics Society." *Journal of the American Geriatrics Society* 60, no. 10 (October 2012): 1957–68. doi:10.1111/j.1532-5415.2012.04187.x.BrightFocus Foundation. "Alzheimer's Disease Research and Education." Accessed March 5, 2017. http://www.brightfocus.org/alzheimers.

Brody, H., L. D. Hermer, L. D. Scott, L. L. Grumbles, J. E. Kutac, and S. D. McCammon. "Artificial Nutrition and Hydration: The Evolution of Ethics, Evidence, and Policy." *Journal of General Internal Medicine* 26, no. 9 (September 2011): 1053–58. doi:10.1007/s11606-011-1659-z.

Buda, O., D. Arsene, M. Ceausu, D. Dermengiu, and G. C. Curca. "Georges Marinesco and the Early Research in Neuropathology." *Neurology* 72, no. 1 (January 6, 2009): 88-91. doi:10.1212/01.wnl.0000338626.93425.74.

Cimons, Marlene. "FDA Approves First Alzheimer's Disease Treatment Medication." *The Tech* 113, no. 40 (September 10, 1993). Accessed February 5, 2017. http://tech.mit.edu/V113/N40/fda.40w.html.

Cleveland Clinic. "Alzheimer's Disease Glossary of Terms."
Accessed March 5, 2017. http://my.clevelandclinic.org/
health/articles/alzheimers-disease-glossary-of-terms.

———. "Hip Fracture." Accessed March 6, 2017. http://
my.clevelandclinic.org/health/articles/hip-fracture.

ClinicalTrials.gov. "Learn About Clinical Studies." Accessed
May 9, 2017. https://clinicaltrials.gov/ct2/about-studies/
learn#ClinicalTrials.

Consumer Reports Health. "Feeding Tubes for People
with Alzheimer's Disease: When You Need Them—
And when You Don't." Accessed March 5, 2017. http://
consumerhealthchoices.org/wp-.

Crossroads Hospice and Palliative Care. "Hospice Care
Guidance: Nutrition at the End of Life." Accessed April
26, 2017. https://www.crossroadshospice.com/caregiver-
guidance/nutrition-hydration/.

Dunn, Hank. *Hard Choices for Loving People: CPR, Feeding
Tubes, Palliative Care, Comfort Measures, and the Patient with
a Serious Illness.* 5th ed. Lansdowne, VA: A & A Publishers,
2009.

Givens, Jane L., MD, MSCE, Kevin Selby, MD, Keith S.
Goldfeld, MPA, MS, and Susan L. Mitchell, MD, MPH.
"Hospital Transfers Among Nursing Home Residents with
Advanced Dementia." *Journal of the American Geriatrics
Society* 60, no. 5 (May 2012): 905–9. doi:10.1111/j.1532-
5415.2012.03919.x.

Hanson, Laura C., Mary Ersek, Robin Gilliam, and Timothy S. Carey. "Oral Feeding Options for Patients with Dementia: A Systematic Review." *Journal of the American Geriatrics Society* 59, no. 3 (March 2011): 463–72. Accessed March 6, 2017. https://www.ncbi.nlm.nih.gov/pmc/articles/PMC3164780/.

Irwin, S., B. T. Mausbach, D. Koo, S. K. Roepke-Buehler, E. A. Chattillion, J. E. Dimsdale, T. L. Patterson, S. Ancoli-Israel, P. J. Mills, R. von Känel, M. G. Ziegler, and I. Grant. "Association Between Hospice Care and Psychological Outcomes in Alzheimer's Spousal Caregivers." *Journal of Palliative Medicine* 16, no. 11 (November 2013): 1450–54. doi:10.1089/jpm.2013.0130.

Kind, Viki. "Avoiding the Pitfalls in CPR/DNR Decision Making." Accessed March 21, 2017. http://kindethics.com/2010/09/10-pitfalls-to-avoid-in-dnr-decision-making/.

Marley, Marie. "Make Alzheimer's End-of-Life Healthcare Decisions Long Before You Need Them," *Huffpost: The Blog.* May 22, 2012. http://www.huffingtonpost.com/marie-marley/alzheimers_b_1436702.html.

Mayo Clinic. "Mild Cognitive Impairment." Accessed March 5, 2017. http://www.mayoclinic.org/diseases-conditions/mild-cognitive-impairment/home/ovc-20206082.

Medline Plus. "Do-Not-Resuscitate Order." Accessed March 6, 2017. https://medlineplus.gov/ency/patientinstructions/000473.htm.

Menzies, Isaura B., Daniel A. Mendelson, Stephen L. Kates, and Susan M. Friedman. "Prevention and Clinical Management of Hip Fractures in Patients with Dementia."

Geriatric Orthopedic Surgery & Rehabilitation 1, no. 2 (November 2010): 63–72. doi:10.1177/2151458510389465.

National Institute of Nursing Research. "Palliative Care: The Relief You Need When You're Experiencing the Symptoms of Serious Illness." Accessed March 6, 2017. https://www.ninr.nih.gov/sites/default/files/Palliative-Care-Relief-When-Experiencing-Symptoms-Serious-Illness-508.pdf.

National Institute on Aging. "Advance Care Planning." Accessed March 21, 2017. https://www.nia.nih.gov/health/publication/advance-care-planning#wishes.

———. "Caregiver Guide: Tips for Caregivers of People with Alzheimer's Disease," PDF, 15. Accessed March 5, 2017. https://www.bu.edu/alzresearch/files/pdf/NIAcaregiverguide03-073.pdf.

———. "Caring for a Person with Alzheimer's Disease: Your Easy-to-Use Guide from the National Institute on Aging," PDF. Accessed March 5, 2017. https://www.nia.nih.gov/sites/.../caring_for_a_person_with_alzheimers_disease_0.pdf.

———. "NIA Timeline." Accessed February 5, 2017. https://www.nia.nih.gov/about/nia-timeline.

———. "Rummaging and Hiding Things: Alzheimer's Caregiving Tips." Accessed March 5, 2017. https://www.nia.nih.gov/alzheimers/publication/rummaging-and-hiding-things.

National Institutes of Health, "The Basics," accessed May 9, 2017, https://www.nih.gov/health-information/nih-clinical-research-trials-you/basics.

Palecek, Eric J., MSIV, Joan M. Teno, MD, MS, David J. Casarett, MD, MA, Laura C. Hanson, MD, MPH, Ramona L. Rhodes, MD, MPH, and Susan L. Mitchell, MD, MPH. "Comfort Feeding Only: A Proposal to Bring Clarity to Decision-Making Regarding Difficulty with Eating for Persons with Advanced Dementia." *Journal of the American Geriatrics Society* 58, no. 3 (March 2010): 580–84. doi:10.1111/ j.1532-5415.2010.02740.x.

PalliativeDoctors.org. "Frequently Asked Questions about Hospice and Palliative Care." Accessed March 6, 2017. http://palliativedoctors.org/faq.

Pearce, J. M. S. "Alzheimer's Disease." *Journal of Neurology, Neurosurgery & Psychiatry* 68, no. 3 (March 1, 2000): 348. doi:10.1136/jnnp.68.3.348.

Sabatino, Charles P. "10 Legal Myths About Advance Medical Directives." Accessed March 13, 2017. http://www.pluk.org/ ITVdocs/PFT_12-03-07_materials.pdf.

Schonwetter Ronald S., MD, B. Han, B. Small, B. Martin, K. Tope, W. Haley. "Predictors of Six-Month Survival Among Patients with Dementia: An Evaluation of Hospice Medicare Guidelines." *American Journal of Hospice and Palliative Medicine* 20, no. 2 (March–April 2003): 105–113. doi:10.1177/104990910302000208.

Shenk, David. "The Memory Hole." *The New York Times* online. November 3, 2006. Accessed May 2, 2017. http:// www.nytimes.com/2006/11/03/opinion/03shenk.html.

Teno, Joan M., MD, MS, Pedro L. Gozalo, PhD, Ian C. Lee, Sylvia Kuo, PhD, Carol Spence, PhD, Stephen R. Connor, PhD, and David J. Casarett, MD, MA, "Does

Hospice Improve Quality of Care for Persons Dying from Dementia?" NIH Public Access Author Manuscript. Accessed May 9, 2017. https://www.ncbi.nlm.nih.gov/pmc/articles/PMC3724341/pdf/nihms480027.pdf.

Triplett, P., B. S. Black, H. Phillips, S. Richardson Fahrendorf, J. Schwartz, A. F. Angelino, D. Anderson, and P. V. Rabins. "Content of Advance Directives for Individuals with Advanced Dementia." *Journal of Aging and Health* 20, no. 5 (August 2008): 583–596. doi:10.1177/0898264308317822.

Urdan, Laurence. *The Bantam Medical Dictionary,* 3rd rev. ed. New York: Bantam, 2000.

US Department of Health and Human Services. "Estimates of Funding for Various Research, Condition, and Disease Categories (RCDC)." NIH Categorical Spending: NIH Research Portfolio Online Reporting Tools. Published February 10, 2016. Accessed March 5, 2017. https://report.nih.gov/categorical_spending.aspx.

Volicer, Ladislav, MD, PhD. "End-of-Life Care for People with Dementia in Residential Care Settings." PDF. The Alzheimer's Association. Accessed March 6, 2017. https://www.alz.org/documents/national/endoflifelitreview.pdf.

Yoneyama, Takeyoshi, DDS, PhD, Mitsuyoshi Yoshida, DDS, PhD, Takashi Ohrui, MD, PhD, Hideki Mukaiyama, DDS, Hiroshi Okamoto, DDS, PhD, Kanji Hoshib, DDS, PhD, Shinichi Ihara, DDS, Shozo Yanagisawa, DDS, Shiro Ariumi, DDS, Tomonori Morita, DDS, Yasuro Mizuno, DDS, Takayuki Ohsawa, DDS, PhD, Yasumasa Akagaw, DDS, PhD, Kenji Hashimoto, DDS, MD, PhD, Hidetada Sasaki, MD, PhD, and Members of the Oral Care Working Group. "Oral Care Reduces Pneumonia in Older Patients in Nursing Homes." *Journal of the American Geriatrics Society* 50, no. 3 (April 2002): 430–33. Accessed March 6, 2017. https://www.researchgate.net/publication/11423562_ Oral_care_reduces_pneumonia_in_older_patients_in_ nursing_homes.

About the Author

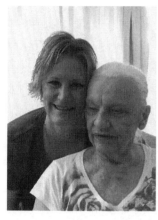

Amy Neuzil's career in healthcare has spanned thirty years. After graduating from nursing school in 1986, she spent her career working as a pediatric nurse, embracing a concept known as family-centered care. As Amy's mom began showing signs of memory loss, she noticed parallels between family-centered care for children and family-centered care for vulnerable adults. Similar to her experience as a young pediatric nurse, with eldercare, family members are the support system and caregivers for their loved ones, whether they are a traditional family or a group of people committed to caring for one another. Since 2004, Amy has worked and volunteered as a licensed massage therapist in healthcare and hospice settings in Cincinnati, Ohio. Additionally, she volunteers at her church, her son's school, and from time to time, at the local chapter of the Alzheimer's Association.

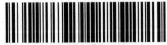

Made in the USA
Lexington, KY
05 September 2017